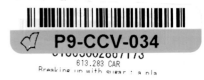

BREAKING UP WITH SUGAR

BREAKING UP WITH SUGAR

A Plan to Divorce the Diets,
Drop the Pounds, and Live Your Best Life

MOLLY CARMEL

AVERY
an imprint of Penguin Random House
New York

AVERY

an imprint of Penguin Random House LLC
penguinrandomhouse.com

Copyright © 2019 by Molly Carmel

Most Avery books are available at special quantity discounts for bulk purchase for sales promotions, premiums, fund-raising, and educational needs. Special books or book excerpts also can be created to fit specific needs. For details, write SpecialMarkets@penguinrandomhouse.com.

Library of Congress Cataloging-in-Publication Data

Names: Carmel, Molly, author.
Title: Breaking up with sugar : a plan to divorce the diets, drop the
    pounds, and live your best life / Molly Carmel.
Description: New York : Avery, an imprint of Penguin Random House, [2019] |
    Includes bibliographical references and index. | Summary: "A proven plan
    to break free from your unhealthy relationship with Sugar - and reclaim
    your health and your life for good"—Provided by publisher.
Identifiers: LCCN 2019030086 | ISBN 9780593086162 (hardcover) |
    ISBN 9780593086179 (ebook)
Subjects: LCSH: Sugar-free diet. | Sugar—Health aspects. | Mind and body.
Classification: LCC RM237.85 .C37 2019 | DDC 613.2/8332--dc23
LC record available at https://lccn.loc.gov/2019030086
p.   cm.

Printed in Canada

10 9 8 7 6 5 4 3 2 1

Book design by Silverglass

To you, my brave reader, for taking *another* chance in the name of the life you deserve. Your perseverance, courage, and hope has kept me relentlessly on the path to try harder, dig deeper, and write this book.

And to my mentor and treasured friend, Dr. Marty Lerner, one of the OGs in our field who has fiercely and fearlessly blazed the path for the treatment of food addiction.

Contents

Breaking Up Is Hard to Do

I can't tell you how thrilled I am—relieved, even—that you found this book. Reading this will be one of the best decisions you'll ever make. Bold? Yes. But time is of the essence, my friend, and we've got things to do; bold and brave is our only option. I'm in the business of helping you break free from the great abuser in your life. . . . Sugar, and I take this proposition very seriously.

Now, let's get to *you*. Let's talk about how Sugar has infiltrated and hijacked your life. I know how much pain, shame, isolation, and suffering this relationship has caused you. I know how hopeless and alone you've felt. I know because I spent many years feeling this way myself, and I now dedicate my life to helping people who know it all too well. I approach this topic—and you—with all my heart and my commitment to help you change your relationship with food, divorce dieting, and create your very best relationship with . . . *yourself.*

How do you know if this book is for you? Have you ever:

- Reached for a quick cookie pick-me-up at three p.m., only to mow through the entire sleeve?
- Intended *not* to not finish the pint of ice cream, yet found yourself licking the carton clean again?
- Promised yourself just one bite of dessert, only to find yourself scouring the kitchen searching for more?

- Left your house late at night to get more of your Sugar-du-jour?
- Felt unsatisfied after having a "normal" portion of cake?
- Had trouble focusing during dinner with your friends because you can't stop thinking about the bread?
- Awoken the morning after a binge feeling sick and full of shame?
- Avoided social situations because you don't feel comfortable in your body and clothes?
- Counted the minutes until your meeting is over so you can get to the vending machine?
- Hidden or lied about how much Sugar you eat?
- Been embarrassed about the range of clothing sizes you have in your closet?
- Had to buy new clothes because nothing you have fits?
- Suffered from insomnia or constantly felt the need to sleep as a result of your eating habits?
- Had a doctor express concern about your health—diabetes, insulin resistance, high liver enzymes, and the like—and not been able to accept or follow recommendations of decreasing your Sugar consumption?
- Stayed home instead of going out with your friends or family because you just wanted to be alone with your Sugar?
- Gotten into arguments with the people you love the most about your weight, health, eating habits, or relationship with Sugar?

Do you find yourself making promises you can't keep about eating Sugar? Eating more of it than you swear you will? Finding it harder than you think it should be to stop? Do you ever hear the voice of Sugar seducing you back in?

You're always so good. You deserve it.
Everyone eats treats sometimes. Don't you just want to be normal?
It's a celebration! Everyone's having so much fun! Don't be a downer.
You can have a little more, no one will know.
This time it will be different.

It's so good! Don't deny yourself pleasure.
Just a bite or two. You'll get back on the wagon tomorrow.
You've already screwed up your diet. Who cares what you eat next?
There's no point in trying to quit; this is just who you are.
Skip the debate, you know you'll eat. Let's get on with it.

As you may already know, the voice gets bolder and more convincing over time, and the behaviors more demoralizing. Help is here. I know you've heard that before, but just hear me out. What you're about to read is unlike anything you've seen before. Pinky swear.

This book is about how to set you free in every way possible—so that you can release the weight that's piled on from day-, week-, year-long binges, add energy to your life, improve your health, connect on deeper levels to those around you, and take greater risks. I want to help the light inside you turn from dim to high voltage. And that's just the short list. Freedom in every area of life awaits you—and I've got your back.

Why me? Well, as the old commercial used to say, "I'm not only the Hair Club president, I'm also a member." Your struggle was my struggle, and my passion for helping you to find your solution comes from the deepest and most personal place: as someone who understands the plight of compulsive overeating and food addiction, who couldn't get help because the right kind of help didn't exist. I battled my food and weight disorder—tipping the scales at 325 pounds—for more than twenty years before I found hope. Much more about this in the next chapter. Suffice it to say, it was bumpy, muddy, and filled with tragedy until finally I was able to piece together a recovery and find a way to create the help I needed. I heard a voice inside my head when I was thirteen years old and attending a weight-loss camp in Connecticut. It said, "You should help people. You should make a program that works." So I did—amassing degrees, participating in trainings, reading literature, going outside the lines of what traditional fields of psychology, addiction, and nutrition said was right. I opened the doors to my Manhattan clinic, the Beacon, in 2012. Thousands of clients later, I've never looked back. And now I'm here, in a place I've always dreamed of—excited, but mostly humbled and honored to be your guide.

So what's on the proverbial menu? First, we're going to talk a bit about your relationship history and get down to one of the key reasons you can't find the peace and freedom you need. Then we're going to dive in and learn the real truth about your great love, Sugar—the ins and outs, the ups and downs. With science by our side, we are going to decide whether it's time for a breakup. If it is, we are going to map out the life that you want and deserve, shed some tears, have a grieving ceremony, and kick Sugar to the curb once and for all. I'm going to outfit you with a meal plan that will keep you full and that will fit into your life—restaurants, travel, spur-of-the-moment plans—yes, yes, yes! I'm going to give you some guidelines—66-day vows—to abide by to help you get the results you deserve. I'm going to teach you a whole new set of skills so that you're not turning to Sugar when times get tough, thwarting all your amazing progress. We're going to create solutions for the roadblocks no one talks about—what to do when the binge is on and what to do when you don't want to do what you know you should do. I'm going to teach you how to reduce the harm and not make bad situations worse. We're going to break you free of your unhealthy relationship to Sugar—we're going to bust you out of the prison you're in.

And then I'm going to teach you how to be in an honest and loving relationship with food and with yourself. Because in some ways, breaking up is the easy part. Sort of. You've quit a lot of things before. It's the staying broken up that's tough. In order for you to stay away from Sugar, we're going to have to dissolve one more relationship so that you completely repair your relationship with food; you're going to have to *divorce dieting*. You're going to learn how to be committed through the messy spells and tough times, so that you can break your current patterns of mass destruction when things get tough. Our endgame is to keep you on the road to (mostly) fabulous, forever.

I'm going to teach you how you can stop cutting and running back to Sugar. Imagine if you gave up every time you made a mistake in your marriage, friendships, or work relationships—think about what you would lose if you sacrificed an entire relationship every time things got tough. The secret to this new, beautiful relationship is just that—to treat it *as a relationship*, with the love, patience, and perseverance with which you do all the other worthwhile things in your life.

My favorite piece of data says that real change comes from self-determination—it's the single most important factor that determines whether a change will stick. The science tells us that people who have internal motivation—like improving health or increasing happiness—and are determined *for themselves* to accomplish their goals are more likely to be successful in changing their behavior. In short, that means this breakup, this new life, has to be completely *yours*—and by the end of this book, you will have created a unique and amazing relationship with food and with yourself, and crafted a road map for a life that is sweeter and more satisfying than any cookie, cake, or candy. Double pinky swear.

This freedom is very possible. I've found it myself and I have witnessed thousands of people successfully break up with Sugar. They are flourishing and so can you. Imagine your life with a completely neutral relationship with Sugar. The cravings don't control you—you sit at meals, gatherings, parties, enjoying conversations and life around you, not plagued by if and when Sugar is going to return to rule the roost. Because of the new relationship you're going to create, you'll be able to experience a new kind of peace when it comes to food. You'll focus on eating when it's time to eat, but mostly you'll focus on the more exciting things in your life. It's *you* who will have the power—not the Sugar cravings. You'll remain one size, never worrying about whether clothes are going to fit or pants are going to split a seam. You have the ability to focus on things you never thought possible—new relationships, new passions. And, most important, you'll have a loving, trusting, compassionate, and confident relationship with *yourself*, the most critical relationship of all.

All this is yours for the taking. You've heard about your best life. Now it's time to live it.

Part 1

The Intervention

Chapter 1

My Breakup with Sugar

My name is Molly, and I was in a horribly abusive relationship with Sugar.

If ten years ago you had told me, a leading eating disorder and addictions therapist, that my relationship with Sugar was abusive, that I was actively and dangerously addicted to Sugar and had been for nearly thirty years, I would have told you that you were crazy.

I would have told you that fat was the problem, that leptin was the problem, that genetics were the problem, that anything *but* Sugar was the problem. What I would have sworn, what had infiltrated my deepest belief system, was that *I was the problem*. Because abusers can become that powerful, and because addicts protect their substances, I would have told you that a life without muffins, candy corn, oatmeal raisin cookies, French bread, and angel hair pasta was not a life worth living.

Even with the demoralizing binges in which Sugar was always the main player, even with the terrible and life-threatening weight gain, even with my loved ones expressing serious concern about my weight and behavior, even with the desire to isolate myself with my favorite foods, even with waking up many mornings with a Sugar-related hangover, even with the constant guilt and shame stemming from my behavior with food, even with my never-ending feelings of self-loathing, I still would have told you that breaking up with Sugar wasn't an option.

Sugar soothed me! It helped me unwind after a long day! Sugar was the fun at the party! It was an integral part of my social life. Everyone overeats from time to time, right? Everyone gets sick from Halloween candy or overindulging in dessert. It's *no big deal.*

I thought Sugar was my solution, when all along it was really my problem. It controlled me in ways I was simply unable to see. And when I *could* see it, I thought I might die if I had to end my relationship with Sugar. Sounds a whole lot like an abusive relationship, doesn't it?

As it turns out, I've been a Sugar addict from the very beginning. I've struggled with my weight since I was born. At nine pounds, twelve ounces, I already had the biology of a big-boned gal and the genetically obese family tree to back it up.

My father died tragically in a car accident a few weeks shy of my third birthday, and when I, at the age of four, began to understand that loss, Sugar became my great love. That's where our relationship truly began. Sugar was my go-to: to soothe, to numb, to feel included, for fun, for enjoyment, for excitement, for passion, for nurturing. And unlike some of the players of my tumultuous childhood, Sugar always showed up for me—it was reliable and never let me down.

The obsession began, and with that, so did Sugar's inevitable hold on me. It was my everything: When my family said we were going to the amusement park, I didn't care about the rides or the games. I was most excited by the cotton candy and funnel cakes. I looked forward to "homework" time at my friend Jenny's house, where I knew the M&M's and coffee cake were plentiful. Middle school lunchtime found me sprinting to the fifty-cent cafeteria "big cookies." Never having been a one-serving-and-I'm-satisfied kind of eater, I found the cravings and quantities of food got bigger and bigger, my deep love and obsession of all things Sugar got more serious, and my weight began to skyrocket.

Every adult in my life was concerned about my weight and my infatuation with food. When I was seven, my mother took me to a leading hospital's nutrition program. I learned about portion sizes and moderation, and got coloring books to try to help me with my weight problem. Even at that age, I knew for sure that the idea of moderation was simply impossible for me. Most of my encounters with food were of the "it's not enough" or "how much more can I have" variety. When it came to Sugar, the stop valve in my brain did not work. Having a normal serving of cake at a friend's birthday party and feeling satisfied was not in my wheelhouse. I always wanted more.

A sliver of cake? That's a good one, nutritionists! And still, I tried—with all my might—to be okay with the sliver, to have the "healthy portion." Epic fail each and every time. The sliver led to sneaking a little more, which led me to endless stomachaches after birthday parties, and still, always wanting more Sugar. As we continued to try the hospital program, my mother instituted the suggested rules, which resulted in me finding more creative ways to get my Sugar. I started trading food with friends at lunch, sneaking treats from the cupboards of my house when my mom wasn't watching, and taking quarters and dollars out of the pockets of coats in my house to get cookies and candy at school.

Suffice it to say, that program was not effective. All it really did was solidify my passion and love for Sugar. By the time I was ten years old, I was willing to go to great lengths and act against my value system in the name of Sugar.

My experience at that hospital program was the beginning of a long career as a chronic and failed dieter. There were a multitude of miserably failed nutritionists, weight-loss camps, and a litany of diet programs—typical and atypical—that would follow.

A few attempts did lead to some success, but these "successes" were the most disheartening of all. When a cat kills a mouse, it doesn't kill it in one fell swoop. It plays with it. Tortures it. The cat will attack the mouse, and then release it and let it run around a little, letting the mouse believe it's been freed from the jaws of death. In this moment of peace, the cat attacks once again. The same can be said about me and Sugar—Sugar was the cat and I was the mouse.

At eleven, I was the youngest person at the Weight Watchers meetings. I proudly lost nine pounds before the Sugar took over. I started to lie in my WW journals and then just stopped writing entirely. I would fake sick before the meetings or make playdates when I knew it was time for weigh-in. Sugar: 1; Weight Watchers and Molly: 0.

By fourteen, I was relegated to summer weight-loss camp. Sadly, I knew in the bottom of my heart that even if I was successful, I was going to come home and gain all my weight back, which I inevitably did. Another score for Sugar.

High school was a blur of Weight Watchers meetings followed by gorging at the diner; purchasing over-the-counter diet pills and chasing those with cupcakes and milkshakes; making empty promises to countless nutritionists; attempting acupuncture; earnestly trying the Atkins diet as well as *Stop the Insanity!* and eating low-fat with Susan Powter; willingly drinking SlimFast shakes; and ordering Jenny Craig and Nutrisystem—only to find myself rebounding from all those programs with piles of spaghetti and sleeves of cookies. Sugar was my master, once again.

By my senior year, I was tipping the scales at 225 pounds, buying my 3X prom dress from a catalog because there weren't stores in those days that catered to plus-sized prom goers. While my friends excitedly showed off their slinky, tight-fitting black-tie dresses that they absolutely adored, I was crossing my fingers that my dress would fit and praying I could look remotely acceptable. More demoralization, more shame.

It never, ever occurred to me to call this problem an addiction, or to say that I was engaged in an abusive relationship with Sugar. But that's exactly what it was. Time and time again, full of hope, I would attempt another diet program. Little did I know, I was bringing a knife to a gunfight—these programs were completely outmatched by my abusive relationship with Sugar and the hold it had on me.

Diets always failed me and, quite frankly, I wound up in an abusive and addictive relationship with them just like I did with Sugar. I was infatuated with the promises, the quick fixes, the goal weights, the before and after pictures. I strived to be their poster child. There was no diet I wouldn't try—no guarantee I wouldn't believe to help heal my pain and obesity. And there was no plan that ever fulfilled its vow to me.

I thought that each new diet would be different—that this time it would work. I always ended up failing, and I became more miserable and heavier than when I had begun. And worse than that, I found myself embedded in deep self-hate, feeling certain that something was wrong with *me*—that I was bad, defective, and weak because no matter how hard I tried, I couldn't get better.

I became a certified aerobics instructor—in hopes that the title would help keep me trim and sustain some of the weight loss I had achieved at camp that year. I had a period of maintaining my weight in college via very low-fat eating, calorie counting, working out, and teaching aerobics two or three times a day. I can remember waking up at the crack of dawn to get my morning workout in, putting vinegar on my salads, and being utterly terrified of regaining the weight. Of course I was going to regain it! And so it went: My friends found a fat-free frozen yogurt shop, and weekly outings for them became daily outings for me. Smalls became mediums became larges with toppings. Before I knew it, I was sleeping through my workouts. Sugar was back in charge, running the show, and I was home alone, eating in an unmanageable way, too ashamed to go out in clothes that no longer fit. With that weight gain, I was fired from my job at the aerobics studio. They told me they were getting too many complaints about my size and ability to keep up with the class.

As with most stories of abuse and addiction, my relationship with Sugar got much, much worse before it got better. I hit very scary, dark, and lonely bottoms. My addiction to Sugar and resulting obesity impacted every single part of my life.

I moved to Ann Arbor, Michigan, for graduate school and had to drop out because my relationship with Sugar became so toxic and severe. I essentially ate my way through my time there, topping out at over 325 pounds.

By now, the relationship impacted me physically: It caused medical problems—severe migraines, reflux, eczema, exhaustion, and excruciating joint pain. I was morbidly obese, the evils of which only those who have experienced it can really understand: agonizing skin chafing, unbearable lower back pain, intense odors. I stopped being able to tie my shoes and literally had to squeeze into my relatively small shower. Seat belt extenders and the shame of not fitting into things—airplane seats, elevators, restaurant booths, amusement park rides—became the norm.

Buttons were popping off my blouses, my pants were splitting down the middle, my neck and wrists had gotten so big that I could no longer wear my jewelry; I stopped wearing underwear and bras because they had become too small. It came time to surrender completely to plus sizes for all my clothing. This was back in a day before internet shopping, when there were only two stores that served plus-size women.

As in so many abusive relationships, my relationship with Sugar caused me to isolate myself; the shame and depression of my weight was too much for me to handle and too painful for me to share with anyone else. Sugar was there to help numb these feelings. Unbeknownst to me, I was deep in the cycle of addiction and abuse. It would be a guaranteed "no" when friends asked me to go out. I stopped having fun—no movies or concerts—I was too tired, too scared I wouldn't fit into the seats, too self-conscious that people would make fun of my weight. I wouldn't even visit my beloved grandparents in California. I feared their judgment and the judgment of others as I tried to wedge myself into an airplane seat. I struggled with prejudice and discrimination, which left me utterly depressed and defeated.

I used Sugar to make me feel better. It did for a short time, but it was only temporary. The feelings would come back and I'd have to use more Sugar to escape it—Sugar was my solution *and* my problem. I was stuck in this endless cycle with no way out.

I saw countless psychiatrists and therapists; read books; went to acupuncturists, ashrams, and hospitals; and took numerous psychotropic medications—all in the name of defeating this shame, depression, and weight gain. Sugar was the cause and I was trying to use it as my cure. All along I would have told you that something was wrong with *me*. That I wasn't enough, that I was deficient, that I didn't have the willpower, that I was cursed, a loser, unlovable, fat for life.

I was breaking an almost daily promise to myself to try to get help and get better. Pair this with years of repeated diet failure, constant stigmatization because of my weight and size, chronic depression, and physical pain. *This is the recipe to kill a spirit.*

In 2000, my grandmother saw Carnie Wilson talking to Oprah about her gastric bypass surgery. She demanded I get it. She was scared

I was going to die, and that was most certainly the path I was walking. So I went under the knife and got my intestines rerouted. Of course I did! I was at my bottom, or at least what I thought was my bottom. Though it felt aggressive to do something so permanent and intense, I also felt like I was out of options and would do anything to get out of the excruciating physical and psychic pain. I believed the surgery might be the answer to my prayers—that it just might fix everything.

Naturally, that's not how the story goes. While I lost some weight, that weight loss came with great consequences. I acquired a serious case of bulimia that annihilated my teeth and esophagus, which caused my friends to intervene, and I exacerbated an alcohol addiction that I would have to recover from in the years to come.

Less than two years after the surgery, surprise! I was right back in the middle of the chaos and self-hate of my abusive relationship with Sugar—bingeing on bagels and pizza and ice cream, gaining weight and struggling with near-suicidal depression.

When I was at my first weight-loss camp, knowing that I was going to come home only to be demoralized by regaining all my weight, a little voice inside me screamed: *"You should help people! You should create a program that really works!"* That voice screamed to me during each and every failed attempt at dieting and weight loss. After it became apparent that my bypass was another failed attempt, I went on a quest to find *my* personal solution, while simultaneously going on a professional quest to become qualified to help you find *yours*.

My professional journey led me to extensive training and relative success in the field of behavioral weight management. When I was twenty-five, I moved to California to start the first-ever therapeutic boarding school for adolescent obesity. It was my dream job—I thought I would be able to help kids in a way that had never been available to me.

The main focus of the program was low-fat eating, calorie restriction, and exercise—all ideas, I know today, that do not make for a sustainable solution. In the years to come, I ran several very successful programs and was a living example of the benefits of low-fat eating. But you know the story by now: I was living a double life, held prisoner to my abusive relationship with Sugar. I talked the talk and walked the walk—even though that walk led me straight to the oversize tray of fat-free brownies and many late-night binges on cereal, candy, and fat-free muffins.

I was able to maintain a size 12 or 14, largely because I was having much of my food portioned for me at the programs I was running and followed a religious and extreme exercise regime, trying to work off everything I overate, which is one of the hallmarks of bulimia. But I lived in *constant fear* of gaining weight. Sugar addiction hides in every shape and size, and though the pain of morbid obesity was excruciating, the fear of gaining weight after having been morbidly obese may have been worse. While I thought I had figured it out, like the cat with the mouse, Sugar was always in the wings waiting for me—taking any chance it could get to weasel back in with full force.

This relationship with Sugar was very seductive—it would tell me all the time, "Everything is fine. It's the *fat* that is killing you. You and I are fine—great, even. Now pass the Sour Patch Kids." I *loved* Sugar, so I believed the rationalizations. I later discovered that the word *rationalize*, when broken down, is *rational lies*. That applied to me: Anytime someone talked to me about Sugar and the evils it brought, I would refer to them as a "low-carb lunatic" and continue to tout my low-fat lifestyle and that of the programs I was running.

I moved back to New York and began running programs there. Living without the portioned food and constant exercise that had been part of my life in California resulted in an almost fifty-pound weight gain. I was in a *panic*, scared that this weight gain would impact my job, just like it had in college at the aerobics studio, and certain that the 50 pounds would turn into 80, 100, 150 in no time as it had so many times before.

And I saw this happening with my clients. Many of the people I counseled with low-fat choices were not finding real success. They were gorging on jams, Swedish Fish, fat-free brownies, cereal, and pretzels—all seemingly "legal" low-fat foods, but all laden with more Sugar than I can even bear to think about today. And like me, once they started, they couldn't stop. They were coming into my programs, trying to lose weight, trying to follow the prescription I had been trained in, yet they were failing miserably. Something had to be done, and the screaming voice inside me grew louder and louder. *I had to do something.*

Though I had experienced weight loss with a focus on low-fat and calorie restriction, I was also trained with a specialty in addictions, so a part of me knew that my behaviors around food, even while I maintained a lower weight, weren't healthy. I was still obsessed with Sugar—craving it, hiding it, rationalizing it, fighting my intense urges for more-more-more, and ultimately giving in to its seduction with no ability to stop.

Sugar was still in the picture, and because of that, my addiction had full rein. One day in the office break room, I inhaled three low-fat muffins, eating them so quickly that I needed to throw them up. The owner of the clinic, a highly regarded eating disorders doctor, walked in on me purging in the bathroom and asked me in a pointed email, "Do you need to talk to someone about what I just saw?" "I'm fine. I'm on top of it. The food went down the wrong pipe. Thanks for your concern," I replied. Lies, lies, lies—and again, as usual, me protecting my substance. Who had I become?

In that moment I had clarity that I needed to get some real help. Out of ideas, I begrudgingly began attending a fellowship for people who struggle with food. In those rooms I found love, support, and understanding that healed me in ways for which I can never fully express proper gratitude. Sadly, those groups did not specifically help me with my food issues, as all members make their own decisions about what works best for them. There were people in the meetings, though, who would talk about being "Sugar addicts" and not eating Sugar and Flour. I would shake my head at these people, labeling them too restrictive, too fanatical, insane people as far as I was concerned. Maybe *they* needed this kind of intervention, but not me—I was fine. That wasn't my problem. Hysterically crying in a support group, gaining weight hand over fist, but I was fine. Sugar still had its hold on me.

Luckily, I began spending time with a wonderful woman, Amy, who didn't eat Sugar or Flour but was very peaceful and pragmatic about it—basing it on a lot of science, with an easy assuredness that she was addicted to both. In fact, it seemed not eating Sugar and Flour made her life a whole lot easier. While I thought she was a loony zealot, some of what she was saying truly resonated with me. When we would go to dinner, she would pass on the bread, eating joyfully and without any chaos. I, on the other hand, frantically gorged on the fat-free rolls, wishing the pieces were bigger or that Amy would go to the bathroom so I could have just a little more without feeling judged.

At the same time, my brother Mikey and my friend George, who both had long-time weight struggles, started the new Paleo diet fad—which I inaccurately understood as no sugar, no grains. Again, I thought they were crazy. But, as you know, I did love a fad diet. When I saw their results, the abused diet addict in me was awakened, and I challenged myself to try it, at least for a week, and see what happened. I detoxed *hard*— irritability, sweats, exhaustion, cravings like mad. The addictions therapist in me woke up again. This wasn't just a rough time I was having from starting a fad diet. I was *actually* detoxing, like I'd seen so many of my clients go through with alcohol and drugs. I began researching and stumbled upon Dr. Robert Lustig's talk on Sugar addiction, "Sugar: The Bitter Truth." This presentation was starting to gain some real traction, and the medical field was beginning to talk about Sugar addiction as a real and diagnosable illness. Finally, the aha moment, which I didn't know I needed so desperately, had arrived. *I was addicted to Sugar.*

I was war-torn: beat up by this battle with food and weight that I had been waging for so long. And I knew my days of fighting were numbered. I was carrying more weight than was comfortable or good for me, and was straight-up exhausted by the constant worry around my weight and health. My career had been built on helping people release weight and keep it off, and I was silently struggling with it every single day. All I wanted was some peace and quiet—days no longer filled with obsession, struggles, and losing battles. Days where I could feel neutral about food and weight and my body. I didn't even care about feeling great in my skin—I simply wanted to stop the madness.

Inevitably, I knew that if I was going to go into recovery from this addiction of mine—if I was going to be able to leave this abusive relationship I'd had with Sugar for nearly thirty years—my next relationship with food and weight was going to have to be loving and sustainable *and* keep me at a healthy weight. I wanted sanity with my vanity. This desperation allowed me to become open and willing, and to humbly take my breakup with Sugar seriously. As unbelievable as it might sound, for the most part, I haven't eaten Sugar since.

I started telling people that I'd made this life choice, so I'd be accountable and less tempted when Sugar came around and tried to entice me back into the abusive relationship. I would say to myself, "I'm not going to eat sugar today." Little by little, one day became ten days, which then became sixty, and so on. I was totally *in awe* of how possible it was to release weight, keep it off, and be free from the constant urges and Sugar cravings that had been gnawing at me my entire life.

Before, when I lost weight and kept it off, it had never, ever felt sustainable. In fact, it was quite the opposite. I always felt like I was keeping the monster at bay. In some ways, being thinner and harboring the fear of gaining my weight back was far worse than being obese and suffering those effects. At any time, on any given day, in a split second, I could be elbow deep in my abusive relationship with Sugar, the weight coming back at me like a bullet train. When I decided to break up with Sugar, it felt as though the weight of the world had been lifted off my shoulders. Prior to that, my life was black and white. Now I could see color.

With my powerful experience in hand, I knew I had to bring the idea of breaking up with Sugar to the Beacon, my clinic in Manhattan. I was still touting the idea of low-fat eating, and I knew I had to overhaul my program completely. I also knew I needed some reinforcements, which were going to be difficult to find. This may come as a surprise to you, but the eating disorder community is very attached to the idea of moderation in all things and the idea of "intuitive eating." They believe that you can listen to your body's hunger and fullness cues to eat your "trigger foods" with balance and composure and without priority on releasing unnecessary weight. And while this might work for some, I was certain of one thing: *These concepts did not, could not, and would never work for me or the clients I treat.*

Trying to find colleagues—especially nutritionists—who were on board with an addictions-based treatment model felt impossible. Along my research path, I met Dr. Marty Lerner and his staff at Milestones in Recovery in Florida, one of the only inpatient facilities that treat binge eating and eating disorders with an addictions model.

That's where I met the first nutritionist I ever liked, then ultimately came to love and trust with every part of my being: Nikki Glantz. Nikki is a pioneer in the world of food-addiction treatment. Although she was academically and professionally trained in the traditional methods of dietetics and nutrition, something about the moderation and intuitive model of eating recovery didn't resonate with her. In her early career, she would counsel clients by prescribing the food plans she had been taught to utilize, and those clients would stay sick. She had always dreamed of helping people change their unhealthy habits from the ground up, and instead found herself doling out food plans that repeatedly failed her clients. She felt powerless and unmotivated.

A random temp job at Milestones changed her entire life. And mine. And hopefully yours. When she was introduced to this cutting-edge model of eating, Nikki jumped on board, motivated largely by the amazing outcomes of the clients she was treating. Today she remains a guardian in support of helping people to break free of their abusive relationships with Sugar. She has since become a card-carrying member of my Power Circle and my co-contributor to your 66-day food plan.

I was able to bring the idea of *Breaking Up with Sugar* into Beacon, and train my staff in how to end clients' battles with Sugar addiction. Just as I had anticipated, the vast majority of my struggling clients who were gorging on fat-free foods broke out of their abusive relationships with Sugar and found the very same peace and freedom that I had felt in my breakup.

I continue to watch this miracle happen at Beacon on a daily basis. The pleasure I derive and gratitude I feel from helping others to find the answer to this problem is beyond my ability to describe. I am living my dream—and, I believe, my destiny—when I go to work every day and help people to find their rightful solution to their weight issues, end their abusive relationships with Sugar, and discover the happier, healthier, long-term relationship with food that they deserve.

Being morbidly obese and unknowingly trapped in an abusive relationship with Sugar is a pain I wouldn't wish upon my worst enemy. It is an unparalleled recipe for shame and self-hate. I wasted so many years walking around believing that I was the problem: that if I had more commitment, more willpower, if I just tried a little harder, I would release the weight.

I was going from diet to diet agreeing with the delusion that I was a failure. That couldn't have been further from the truth. I wasn't failing the diets; the diets were failing me. I didn't have the right solution to the problem—the solution I am offering you today. Diets focused only on the food and the end goal of weight loss, but they failed to take me step-by-step through each day, through each obstacle, to get to my real end goal. Diets told me what and how much to eat, but not what to do when I just didn't feel like following the plan. Diets failed to address the subtle thinking patterns and behaviors that interfered with my ability to "stick to it" for more than a week or two. Diets failed to address the sheer impossibility of self-care and nutrition when I hated and blamed myself for each unsuccessful attempt at releasing weight, viewing myself as the problem and slowly chipping away at my self-worth. Most important, diets failed to correctly identify the specific abuser and addictive substance with which I struggled and that held me captive: *Sugar.*

Which brings me to the next step in my breaking up with Sugar journey: divorcing dieting. I was deep in the binge-restrict cycle—eating enormous quantities of food at night, followed by trying to starve it off come morning. A trusted friend recommended I see Lisa, a nutritionist she knew and respected. While Lisa's plan didn't end up being my exact solution, she taught me some of the fundamentals that inevitably formed my food foundation. She taught me the value of planning my meals ahead of time, of meal regulation—eating every three to four and a half hours a day, four times a day.

That part was not easy. When Lisa suggested that I have yogurt, nuts, *and* fruit for breakfast, I accused her of not understanding my goals. I was certain her suggestion was just going to cause me to binge earlier in the day and gain more weight. She looked me square in the eye and said, "A balanced breakfast is not what is making you fat, Molly. It's the five thousand calories you're bingeing on at night." With that, a lightbulb went off.

One day soon after, I strayed from the food plan Lisa had given me by thoughtlessly grabbing a handful of nuts. My first thought was to head to the convenience store and pick up some ice cream and cookies—I had gone off the plan, so why not go off in style? I remember thinking to myself: *This handful of nuts is certainly not how 'all this' went down. I wonder what would happen if I just got right back on my plan.* And I did. Without the big dramatic binge and discouraging crawl back to the next diet. Just right back on my plan. Business as usual.

This was a pivotal moment for me: I realized Sugar wasn't the only thing holding me captive. There was also the black-and-white, good-or-bad, on-or-off toxic and rigid way I approached my food, left over from years of destructive dieting. After giving up Sugar, I still had more work to do to create a lasting relationship with food. *I had to divorce dieting.* Divorcing dieting didn't mean that I declared a free-for-all, giving in to cravings when they came to haunt me. Quite the opposite: It meant committing to my new relationship, managing the difficulties—and figuring out what worked and what didn't. It meant learning about myself and my food, and staying the course as the relationship grew and flourished. And it's flourished beyond what I could have imagined, *ever.*

My story of Sugar addiction and compulsive dieting is just that, mine. Yours may look and sound completely different, which doesn't mean you aren't a slave to Sugar, too. Maybe you don't struggle with morbid obesity and can't relate to seat belt extenders or plus-size clothes. Maybe you haven't had medical problems associated with your weight or food behaviors . . . yet. If you're not relating, it may be the case that your Sugar-addicted mind is reading my story and already scheming to find a way to have its cake and eat it too (literally). These lies and rationalizations are the hallmark of addiction, and they keep us from the big beautiful life we all deserve. If you're not sure, there is a whole chapter of this book dedicated to helping you gain clarity on where you fall on this scale (you can check that out, come chapter four).

Sugar addiction comes in all shapes and sizes, in all stories, in all bodies. If you find yourself deep into a box of doughnuts—again—when you've *sworn* to yourself you wouldn't, you probably have a problem with Sugar. If you find yourself in the kitchen finishing off a loaf of bread or your kids' animal crackers, hoping no one wakes up to hear you, you are probably in an abusive relationship with Sugar. If you are successful in so many parts of your life, yet cannot "succeed" at eating Sugar in moderation, then you know how it feels to be addicted to Sugar. This isn't about self-control or discipline; this is about Sugar. And regardless of how your food problems look on your body—overweight, "normal" weight, or underweight—you do not deserve to live in a constant state of fear, shame, and self-loathing because you can't "control" yourself around food.

Maybe you're not overweight, maybe you're managing this relationship by over-exercising or starving yourself so you can get your fix without it showing, maybe you only *occasionally* worry about this relationship, maybe you're living a life in which starting over is the norm and freedom feels impossible. The point is: You relate. And that is why I've written this book. That is why I've dedicated my life to helping people find freedom from that suffering, whether it lives on your body in the form of excess weight or deep inside your heart and soul.

Good news! You're in the right place. You're not alone, there is a solution, and you've found the support you need. Even though it might be super scary, please stick around and keep reading. I'll help you figure out where you are in this relationship and what to do next to live freely. Don't give up yet, okay?

As Albert Einstein said so brilliantly, "We can't solve problems by using the same kind of thinking we used when we created them." You need help. People who come to me for help are among the most amazing, smart, savvy, and successful people I've ever met. Abuse and addiction do not care how rich you are, how intelligent you are, how funny you are, how caring you are—and you are. Despite your best qualities, it's an equal-opportunity epidemic, and one with a solution.

Breaking up with Sugar is the single best decision I have ever made in my life. Being free of this abusive relationship has not only given me my life back, it's given me a better, more fulfilling one than I could have ever imagined. It's worth the work.

My relationship with food today is everything I hoped it would be—peaceful and easy. I don't worry about being too hungry, overeating at meals, or if I should go to the convenience store for a nightly binge run. I feel zero shame about food and I live a full, busy, and generally awesome life. I go out to dinner, go on vacation, eat at cocktail hours, attend weddings, visit my relatives, go to luncheons, and attend all sorts of parties with ease. I have learned what and how much to eat in all these situations, so I can seamlessly participate and engage in all the opportunities and adventures that come with a big life, while maintaining a style of eating that nourishes my body, mind, and spirit.

And I am incredibly satisfied with the food I put into my body, maintaining a healthy weight naturally and without the constant seduction, mind games, and struggle that were a mainstay in my destructive relationship with Sugar and dieting.

This breakup has also given me a relationship with myself rooted in trust and integrity. And as someone who for almost thirty years lived with the broken promises and harmful behavior we all know too well, being in a reliable and loving relationship with myself today is nothing short of a miracle. Breaking up with Sugar has given me a life filled with excitement, love, and hope. Most important, it's one in which I can be dedicated to helping you break free of *your* toxic relationship with Sugar.

I have watched thousands of my clients break up with Sugar and as a result find freedom, success, joy, and happiness in their lives that they didn't know was possible. I'm excited—and, frankly, honored—to help you find the same.

You never have to feel this hopeless, broken, defective, guilty, or shameful again. Ever. If this relationship has held you hostage and stolen from you for far too long, then it's time to break it off and be free of your abusive relationship with Sugar. It's time for you to discover the happier, healthier, long-term relationship with food that you deserve.

I Broke Up with Sugar

Ben

Before I broke up with Sugar, I felt hopeless and trapped, like I was living in a prison of my own making without a solution. At thirty years old, I was eating myself to death; I'd surrendered to this abusive relationship that was destroying me, mind, body, and soul. Though I kept it to myself, I considered my life effectively over and not worth living. As time went on, I spent less time with the people I love and lost my enthusiasm for hobbies and activities I'd previously enjoyed. Almost every night I hid in my dark room and ate until physical exhaustion mercifully struck. When I looked at myself in the mirror, I saw only a part of myself, dimly, and felt nothing but hatred.

Then I found Molly's program. When I first started, I didn't think that this program, or any program, would work. Molly asked me to pretend I thought it would work—to suspend my disbelief. I don't know how or why, but having nothing to lose, I took a leap of faith. Her logic made sense, so I went with it. Within weeks, I began to feel a sense of hope and purpose I had not felt in years. Having spent the previous years feeling old and weary, I began to remember that life is a blessing to be savored, not an ordeal to be endured. And with that, my love for spending time with my family and friends returned. Old relationships were renewed and new ones, forged. Life started getting better and better. I rekindled my love of hobbies that had been casualties of my abusive relationship with Sugar. I found myself looking forward to waking up in the morning instead of dreading the dawn. Even eating became an infinitely more enjoyable experience! Instead of feeling guilt and shame almost every time I ate, I felt satisfied knowing that I was taking one more small step on the endless road of healing and toward full recovery. To this day, I sometimes weep after dinner because I know it is a healthy meal and the last one of the day.

Physically, I've released over seventy pounds; psychologically and spiritually, I feel liberated. Slowly, I'm learning to accept that which seemed unacceptable my whole life: Life will bring pain but also joy.

I learned to accept pain and use my toolbox of skills instead of turning to food. Because of that, I'm able to experience true joy today. It's safe to say that breaking up with Sugar literally saved my life. More than that, it's made it worth living again. I am filled with hope every day, ever grateful for my Power Circle helping me stay on my path of recovery. Today, when I look at myself in the mirror, I see a free man staring back at me and feel pride.

Chapter 2

The Sacred Vow: No More Cutting and Running

Whether you like it or not, you're always in a relationship with food: You're either working to improve the relationship or you're complicit in its destruction.

Let's focus on the word *relationship.* You're in one with food whether you realize it or not. Food is more than something we eat; it's *personal.* We have emotional attachments to it, we associate it with good times and bad, we talk about our *loves,* our *hates,* our *obsessions.* So it's safe to say we are in a relationship with food—one that can bring us comfort, connection, confidence, and love. Or, one that can be really rough going, turning potentially abusive without us even knowing. Usually, we focus on the really good times, which is why breaking free is not always easy.

I wish I could tell you this breakup will be like a rom-com storyline: Girl realizes she's in an abusive relationship with Sugar. Girl buys book to guide her through breakup. Girl bravely breaks free from Sugar's nasty clutches. Girl falls in love with her new way of living. Girl rides off into the sunset with her newfound relationship with herself and food, excited for the big beautiful life ahead of her. Cue credits.

If we're honest, up until now the story may have gone a little more like this: Girl has crazy night bingeing on Sugar. Girl wakes up feeling demoralized. Girl finds quick-fix-cleanse-juicing-guru-fast-diet-du-jour and buys empty promise hook, line, and sinker. Girl inevitably gets seduced by Sugar, runs back, and is once again taken hostage—ravaging the hopes and dreams she once had. Girl (*again*) single-handedly destroys everything she's wanted and wished for—especially her self-esteem and belief in herself. That's more horror flick than rom-com.

Why do your relationship attempts always end up listed in the "scary movie" section? I have an idea. Do you think "chronic cheater" might be a term you'd use to describe your relationship with food? I do. Try it on for size: You make commitments at the beginning of the day and don't follow through; you hide, sneak, and lie your way into unhealthy predicaments with Sugar; you feel shame, embarrassment, low-self-esteem; your integrity is shot. As a chronic cheater, you've repeatedly strayed from the course. Your expectations of what it takes to be in a healthy and lasting relationship have been corrupted. And by lasting, I mean the long haul, not just the three months needed to take off your weight before you get back together with doughnuts. The diet culture has brainwashed you into believing this should be easy, with high rewards and very little work. As of now, your response to a rough patch in your relationship with food is to blame yourself, set your progress on fire, and cut and run back to Sugar. Something has to change.

Before we get into the nitty-gritty of finding you absolute and lasting freedom, I need you to try a relationship vow on for size. This vow is the most important one of all. It's the *Sacred Vow*. It goes like this:

> *I commit to staying the course in my new relationship with*
> *myself and with food. In good times and bad, in sickness*
> *and in health, through overweight and goal weight, to the*
> *furthest extent. I commit to staying the course with integrity.*
> *I commit to staying in this relationship and to not be swayed*
> *by the newest fad diet, or what may seem easier, softer, or*
> *faster. I commit to staying the course even when it's tempting*
> *to run back into the arms of Sugar.*

Relationships are a long game; they are a marathon, not a sprint. As with all successful relationships, there are days you're raring to go and days you're not. I would be doing you the greatest disservice if I let you begin reading this book thinking your new relationship was going to be a fairy tale. It's going to be deeply freeing and meaningful and will allow you to open up your life in a way you never knew possible. But easy? No, not at first. A Disney fairy tale? Not exactly. But no truly strong and healthy relationship exists without some trials and tribulations along the way.

It's certainly not your fault that you're caught in this fallacy that it should be seamless and easy. The billion-dollar diet industry has led you to believe that if it isn't easy, then it must be your fault—*you* are the problem. That's how they make their money and keep you held captive, just like Sugar. If you finish this book knowing only one thing, know this: You are *not* the problem. *Sugar* is the problem. Breaking up with Sugar is your solution.

Thankfully, there's an answer to this relationship problem. We're going to create a new foundation on which to build the relationship you want and deserve with food. That's why I urge you to take this Sacred Vow. This is a vow to stay committed for the long haul, even when it's hard and especially when you make mistakes. This is a vow to not make bad situations worse.

Like all chronic dieters—and chronic cheaters—you have been taught to throw in the towel after every mistake. That abusive voice tells you, *You failed again. See? You have no self-control. This diet won't work. You're worthless, disgusting, shameful, fat. . . .* That abusive voice cues you to cut and run. It allows you to sabotage your relationship with food and with yourself. But the truth is, you're never really cutting and running. Your relationship with food *and* with yourself are two that you can never outrun.

You may be thinking, *Slow it down! I'm not ready to commit to any vows, let alone something sacred!* And to that I say: Of course! *Of course* you're still coming to terms with the idea of giving up this very complicated relationship. It brought you tremendous physical and emotional pain and anguish, and it brought you equally tremendous comfort, security, numbing, and familiarity. It will take great courage and hard work to get over your toxic relationship. And it's why, this early in the book, I am bringing it up *for your consideration*. Because I need you to start thinking about this early. It's like we're planting a seed—one that I hope will flourish and grow into a long and lasting relationship.

The Sacred Vow allows you to begin reparations for the most important relationship you have: the one with yourself. Staying the course will help prove that you can trust yourself again. That you are reliable, worthy of esteem, and chock full of integrity. Years of dieting and this abusive relationship with Sugar have not only hurt your body, they have deeply damaged your heart and soul. The strength and self-assurance that comes from being empowered in your new life will make you truly unstoppable.

Vow to commit to this new relationship—*especially* through those dark and uncomfortable moments—because it is *this* vow that will change your life forever. Please know that staying the course doesn't mean you will do this perfectly. Quite the opposite. Staying the course means you will work through your missteps and lapses, helping to make your relationship stronger. Staying the course will end the feelings of demoralization, shame, and hopelessness that have been the hallmark of your relationship with food. This is where the real cash and prizes come in. It's your starting point to release your weight for good and to create a peaceful relationship with food. It's where you regain the trust and security in yourself that you lost from years of diet drama and trauma, and years of Sugar's abuse. This is where your freedom truly begins.

I Broke Up with Sugar

Callie

Before I broke up with Sugar, my entire existence was consumed with wretched thoughts of food—what my next meal would be, when I'd eat it, what I wouldn't dare allow myself to eat, and reminders about why I had to exert such control: *lose weight, be thin, be good enough.* I would wake up each morning determined to show myself just how "perfect" and "clean" my food could be, because that's where I derived my value. Fast-forward to each night, my self-restraint would break because of stress, emotion, discomfort, hardship, or anxiety, and food became an escape tactic. I mindlessly numbed any pain through food, often before I even realized that I was feeling badly in the first place.

Some of my worst nightly sugar binges left me immobile, frozen in pain, and steeped in guilt and shame. I've skipped work, commitments with friends, and a friend's entire wedding weekend, all because of the debilitating shame around a particularly bad binge. This cycle left me feeling lost, depressed, ill, confused, and hopeless that I could never break this dirty, secret habit. I had forgotten how to eat and more important, how to take care of myself through proper nourishment. I was ashamed at how sorry I felt for myself, and I was fearful that it would only worsen.

The concept of being addicted to food and needing to break up with Sugar had never crossed my mind, and I felt chills the first time I was told that I was an addict. What felt harsh and foreign to me at first quickly became a truth that made perfect sense. My dirty secret was an addiction indeed, but with this admission came a calming relief that I could recover and heal. There was finally a name for this evil game, and now I was playing smart. Through Molly's lessons and support, I began to practice building self-esteem, discovered skills to stop Sugar in its tracks, and created ways of cultivating calm. Soon, a desire to be an estimable, accountable, self-reliant person with a big life became more attractive to me than any Sugar binge.

Breaking up with Sugar did not feel like a death sentence. It was freeing and empowering. This substance had been contributing to a meek, fearful, shameful life for far too long. Becoming Sugar-free literally freed up space in my mind to discover all the ways I could love myself properly. It wasn't easy and still isn't, but the feeling of putting my self-worth ahead of Sugar and dieting is exhilarating. My days now consist of more deep breathing, positive affirmations, moments of gratitude, and plenty of colorful, nutritious, bountiful food. My meals have gone from being analyzed and criticized to being nourishing and energizing. I relish preparing my meals with care and attention, and I get excited about the flavor and nutrients they provide.

The most important lesson I've learned as I've broken up with Sugar is that my relationship with food and myself is never ending, in the best way. I do not consider what I've had to eliminate from my life to recover from my food addiction a loss; instead, I count the many benefits I've gained: peace of mind, acceptance, patience, freedom, and the chance to live a big life. By following Molly's principles for breaking up with Sugar, you can clear up space in your mind and heart that was previously devoted to negative self-talk and redirect that energy toward joy. You can wake up in the morning bursting with clarity and energy, and go to sleep each night thankful for that day. Molly's expertise can completely shift your behaviors, as it did for me. I thought I was a lost cause when I first stepped into her office, but I had no idea the gift of utter love, attention, and understanding I would soon receive. Breaking up with Sugar showed me how tough I am and how far I can go in the name of radical self-love.

Chapter 3

The Truth About Your Sweetest Love

This may feel a little like an episode of *Maury* or *Jerry Springer*—imagine finding out the person you've loved for so long is stealing from you, cheating on you, and has a secret family of four: *major betrayal*.

And it hurts *bad*. But we're going to heal that pain—I promise. The first step of breaking free from this toxic relationship is to learn the bitter truth about your sweetest love. And remember, we're doing this so that we can solve the problem. Knowledge. Is. Power.

But it feels so goooooood!

I know it. Sugar does feel *so* good. And you're not crazy for loving Sugar—it goes back to your beginnings. The minute you cried and your mother gave you milk to soothe you, this relationship got complicated.

The safety and security of Sugar is a story of survival that actually goes back to way before you, your grandmother, and your great-great-great-great-grandmother were even born. Back to the days of hunting and gathering, before we were waltzing down the aisles of our big box stores, or ordering takeout in thirty minutes or less guaranteed. We knew our fruit was safe to eat by its sweetness—you will never find a berry that is both poisonous and sweet. Back then, we also needed our energy *fast*—and Sugar is the fastest and most easily broken down of all nutrients.

Aside from the ancestral soothing, safety, and security we get from Sugar, we also usually associate it with happiness, celebration, and love.

Your birthday? Cake. Hot summer day? Ice cream. Valentine's Day? Chocolate. Celebration at the office? Doughnuts! You know the drill.

So of course you love Sugar! The problem is, your relationship has taken a nasty turn—Sugar has betrayed you. Let's learn about how this all went down—relying, of course, on science and research to shine the light on your path to freedom.

SUICIDE ON THE INSTALLMENT PLAN

I'm sure this ain't your first diet rodeo, so I'm not going to insult you and go through all the research on why Sugar is bad for you. I'm much more interested in telling you why you can't stop overeating it and how to change that. But I'd be remiss if I didn't spend at least a minute or two talking about how absolutely lethal Sugar is for you, physically. We know it impacts your vanity: weight gain, belly fat, breakouts, skin irritation, wrinkles, aging skin, tooth decay, and hair loss. But Sugar also negatively affects *every single part of your body*.

Some of these harmful effects are more well known than others. Eating sugar has been linked to: inflammation, migraine headaches, anxiety, brain fog, trouble sleeping, weakened eyesight, gum disease, heart disease, increased cholesterol, asthma, suppressed immunity, kidney damage, nonalcoholic fatty liver, overworked pancreas, arthritis, osteoporosis, metabolic syndrome, and leptin resistance. There's even terrifying research showing that Sugar increases the risk of developing certain cancers. And of course, let us not forget Sugar's pièce de résistance, glucose intolerance and diabetes. When we ingest Sugar more quickly than our body can metabolize, it's converted to fat, causing weight gain and a whole host of problematic health conditions. While none of these harmful effects instantly kill you, like a heroin overdose or a grand mal seizure from alcohol withdrawal, Sugar is without a doubt killing you. It's doing so at a much slower rate, which makes it that much more insidious. So then here's the real problem: We continue to eat Sugar *despite* the lethal effects on our body. It's like suicide—just on an installment plan.

If this is all news to you, then welcome and I'm sorry and let's get you broken up with Sugar. If you've been in the same camp as the majority of people, bombarded with this reality more times than you can count, then you're well aware that scientific knowledge alone does very little to help break off your long-standing affair with Sugar. If knowledge *alone* worked, then the diet books and the nutritionists and the degrees and the certifications would have solved your problem already. But they haven't. I'm asking you to make a commitment to stay with me so we can get to the core of the problem and find your permanent solution.

How could Sugar do this to me?

You may be thinking: *How could Sugar do this to me? How did it get this bad? Is it really so bad? Why can my best friend have a bite and walk away from the cupcake while I'm jonesing for a dozen more? I hate Sugar so much for doing this to me! I love Sugar so much. Please pass the cookies. . . .*

It's complicated. That's an understatement. Your relationship with Sugar has gone haywire for a whole host of reasons: the nature of Sugar itself, the nature of your environment, and the nature of *you*. These issues are annihilating your relationship with food and fueling your attachment (and maybe your addiction) to Sugar. No two people are impacted in exactly the same way—you're like a snowflake with your own reaction, vulnerability, and sensitivity. This is what makes the whole concept of addiction so complicated.

We are on the road to a permanent, sustainable solution. I'll remind you of this over and over again, so please don't get discouraged by this idea. Trust me. The first step is to simply become informed about why you're in this boat to begin with. The truth may be painful. Like I've said, I totally have your back on this journey. That's why I'm sharing everything I know with you—so that you can make a decision about your relationship with Sugar that's driven by truth and backed by wisdom.

Sugar on steroids

Look at pictures from the 1950s and you'll see people drinking soda and eating cookies like it's no big deal. And it wasn't, really. What happened? Today, our food is *specifically designed* with highly concentrated Sugar and minimal amounts of fiber and protein. And, because of that, it jolts your system by packing a supersized, superpowered oomph! To put it lightly, our Sugar got turbocharged. It's been suped up and doped up. It's become sugar "on steroids." The Sugary food of our lifetime is definitely not the same as it was seventy years ago. Technically speaking, it activates your brain's reward pathways with an intensity and magnitude that nature never would have dreamed of intending. And you have to wonder about the motives of the food companies that made it that way.

What's more, this new millennium high-potency Sugar food is *everywhere*. It's in places we would expect—cookies, cakes, bread, and candy. It's also *hidden* in our peanut butter, salad dressing, protein bars, sauces, deli meats, tomato sauce, and just about every highly processed food you can get. The truth of the matter is we're eating Sugar—knowingly and unknowingly—all day, every day. Sugar intake per capita in the UK, for example, has more than doubled since 1950 and with that, the obesity rate has quadrupled.

Not to point (more) fingers, but this fancy new potent Sugar not only has a stronger hold on you, it's also BFF with the food industry, which helped to create its "bliss point." What's a bliss point? It's a term, coined by the food industry, that refers to that perfect balance of sweetness, fat, and salt that makes you ignore your feelings of fullness, overeat, and crave processed foods more and more. It's made food manufacturers a whole lotta money. The food we eat today has been designed and manipulated to make eating healthfully and intuitively nearly impossible. It's no wonder so many people struggle with listening to their hunger and fullness cues—the foods we're ingesting are deliberately processed to override that system!

As a result, our taste buds have been trained to crave the sweet, bliss-point foods we are all confronted with at every turn. This is effectively a match made in *hell*. It's no wonder your sweetheart has become your worst nightmare.

Toto, we're not in Kansas anymore

If we've made any mark as a culture, we've wholeheartedly embraced that bigger and faster is better and that more is more. Your exposure to food and food cues is unavoidable. They're all around you. Grocery stores are selling forty thousand more items than they did in the 1990s. And you know all about the convenience of convenience stores. We're far more likely to stop at a 7-Eleven or gas station when we're on the run, and fall prey to the snack food and candy rather than take the time and energy to seek out healthier food. We're quickly ordering things, swiping with urgency, quelling our need for instant gratification. No options are off the table and the only answer is "now." It's a fast-food, fast-pay, fast-eat maneuver completed with a swipe, and off you go. The way we live and eat is the furthest thing from intuitive, so why do we expect our relationship with food to be that way?

Dorothy said it best: ". . . we're not in Kansas anymore." Gone are the days of rising with the sun to tend to the farm, coming in for a sensible, balanced lunch, having some downtime, and retiring at sundown. We are sleeping less, working more, and taking worse care of ourselves as a result. This is bad news for our already muddled relationship with Sugar. In this state, not only are we more susceptible to craving the sweetness, comfort, and instant energy burst that Sugar gives, we are also way more vulnerable to wanting more. Brain-imaging studies clearly show that people who sleep less have greater desire and craving for high-calorie foods. What's worse, they find these foods to be more pleasurable, which only increases Sugar's grip.

And it's not just lack of sleep that makes us eat more, it's also stress. When we're glued to our phones, answering emails, texts, calls, social media comments, our attention is demanded at all times. This causes cortisol, our stress hormone, to kick into overdrive, much like if you were in fight-or-flight mode 24-7. While in the short term, stress can suppress the desire to eat, when your body is under stress for prolonged periods of time (like most of us are), cortisol floods your system, increasing your appetite and motivating you to eat. The research is undeniable—when we are stressed we eat more and inevitably gain weight. And it's not just *any* foods that we crave. Wouldn't you know it—it's the high-Sugar foods that, in the short term, counteract our stress response and boost our mood! An increase in cortisol also decreases the body's production of leptin, the hormone that helps you to feel full. This is a double whammy, making you ridiculously hungry without any net to catch you (more on leptin in a bit). All in all, your stress is making you more stressed . . . and hungry.

Given all we know, of *course* we have a problematic relationship with Sugar and of *course* it dominates us! We're tired and bombarded by unhealthy food, and our brains are unequipped to handle that environment. You might think the answer is more willpower, but it isn't. In fact, willpower is a limited resource. We use it constantly throughout the day—getting ourselves to work, making big and little decisions, fulfilling all our daily obligations, and of course saying no to the cookies. By the end of the day, we're cued for a break, a reward. But we're wiped and so is our willpower. Now is when we're most likely to break that promise we made to ourselves to "be good," and we reignite our affair with Sugar.

So the answer isn't more willpower—you've rocked and exhausted the willpower game. The answer is truly about planning, creating new habits, and mastering skills that help to re-up your willpower when life gets tough.

No wonder you can't stop overeating. *Duh*.

Here's where other weight-loss programs, nutritionists, coaches, conventional diet plans, eating disorder professionals, and the like drop the ball. The main reason you can't stop eating is that Sugar has hijacked your brain. Read again: *hijacked*.

That's a hard pill to swallow—of course it is—especially with the multibillion-dollar diet industry minimizing and confusing this issue to benefit their bank accounts. So I brought along my BFFs science and research to help explain it in the most responsible way I know how.

The first thing science and research tell us is that Sugar is a substance with addictive potential. Studies have shown that Sugar dependence looks exactly like that of other addictive substances like alcohol, cocaine, and opiates in brain, body, and behavior. Tolerance, withdrawal, craving, consuming more than intended, unsuccessful efforts to cut down, continued use despite negative consequences . . . sound familiar? A little like your relationship with Sugar? Whether your yes is a tiny whisper or a scream, you're right. Sugar alters your brain, your nervous system, and your endocrine system—that's effectively your entire body! This is the information that is going to help you make the decision to set yourself on the path to freedom—so stick with me.

Sugar, like other drugs, floods the brain with dopamine, a neurotransmitter responsible for wanting and liking. While dopamine does lead us to feel good (liking), it mostly leads us to seek out (wanting). So when our brain is consistently flooded with dopamine, as it is when we are misusing Sugar, we are more driven to seek out than we are to enjoy. Dopamine also affects our decision-making, memory, and learning centers, effectively training us to seek out Sugar. As is the case with other drugs of abuse, we pursue Sugar despite negative consequences. As you know, the feeling of craving is powerful; it motivates us to choose Sugar again and again, without regard for the harmful effects to our body, self-esteem, and relationships (more on examining the effects of Sugar on your life in the next chapter).

And cravings aren't the only indicator of addiction we see. Rats responded to excessive Sugar intake with bingeing, tolerance, and withdrawal, signs such as chattering teeth, tremors, head shakes, a drop in body temperature, increased anxiety, and depression. All in the name of Sugar! What's more, when the rats withdrawing from Sugar were placed in water, they were less likely to swim or climb out, and more likely to passively float. *They had lost their will to survive.*

My goal is not to have you never experience pleasure again. Quite the opposite! The problem is that with prolonged exposure to Sugar, you're dimming your ability to experience pleasure, which affects all facets of your life. Chances are, you need a lot more Sugar *now* to get the same feeling you had when you had your first bite of ice cream as a kid. That's because as you eat more and more Sugar and your brain floods with more and more dopamine, your dopamine receptors begin to thin out. That means progressively more Sugar is needed to achieve that "this is good" feeling.

So while the common belief is that people who eat lots of Sugar just love it more than other people, the reality is actually the opposite. Now that you have built up a tolerance to Sugar, it affects your brain much less than it does someone who doesn't eat it at all. I've had lots of clients point out to me in amazement that after their breakup with Sugar, fruit tastes like a flavor explosion! I know you may be rolling your eyes, but it's true, I promise. Like you, these are clients who would have never considered the idea of fruit as a treat while still in their abusive relationship with Sugar.

The last piece of this hijacked brain-body puzzle is your endocrine system. Quite simply, with Sugar holding you hostage, your body's ability to sense fullness, or satiety, is severely diminished. Let's get specific: When you eat Sugar, your body floods with insulin, a hormone created in the pancreas. Insulin's job is to regulate your blood-sugar levels and allow Sugar to enter your cells and give you energy. However, when we eat too much Sugar, all that insulin begins to block leptin, the satiety hormone. Leptin tells the brain, "You're full—you've had enough! Now go live your big beautiful life until your next meal." When leptin is blocked time and time again, we become leptin resistant and can no longer feel full. So it makes sense that you keep eating and eating with no end in sight!

To make matters worse, excess insulin triggers your body to stop burning and start *storing* fat. So not only are you stuck in a cycle of overeating, you also are packing on excess fat in the process. I can say for sure that one of the greatest gifts of breaking up with Sugar will be the complete rebirth of your relationship with leptin and insulin. With less Sugar in your body and insulin levels back to normal, you put yourself in a much better position to stop overeating and to release your unnecessary weight. So many of my clients are in absolute awe (I am too) of how much sooner they feel full and that they are satisfied finishing a meal—something they never thought possible. #dreamscometrue

THE TRUTH ABOUT YOUR (SOMETIMES) SAVORY LOVE: GRAIN FLOUR

While your heart is broken reading the truth about Sugar, I'm thinking this is the right time to break the news that this book is not only about Sugar, it's also about Sugar's evil and equally toxic and abusive twin, Grain Flour.

Molly! Why are you bringing my love Flour into this—it's a book about Sugar! Before you make a Molly voodoo doll and start stabbing with gusto, read a little further. I'm not talking about grains—wheat, barley, rice, oats and the like. I'm talking about when those items are **ground down** into Flour. *Your body reacts in the same exact way to Grain Flour as it does to Sugar.*

Why Flour? Let's ask science. The process of making Flour involves grinding, which breaks down the cell structure of the grain. As grain becomes refined into Flour, our body reacts as if we're consuming Sugar. This is best explained by the glycemic index (GI), which measures the effect of food on a person's blood-sugar level. A higher GI rating means a higher blood-sugar spike. For example, table Sugar has a GI of about 68 out of 100. Research has shown that people who eat foods with a higher GI are more likely to report addictive eating, and consumption of high-GI foods has been shown to increase reported hunger while stimulating brain regions associated with reward and craving. That makes all the sense in the world to me, as my top two favorite foods that don't love me back are white bread (GI 70) and baguettes (GI 95).

When the food you eat lacks nutrients, it causes your body to want to keep eating. The grinding process that turns whole grains into Flour strips away many of the essential nutrients and minerals. This allows your already nasty relationship with food to worsen. In a study that compared whole wheat to refined wheat flour, the concentration of essential nutrients decreased as the wheat flour became more refined. Even more striking, as a result of the grinding process itself, which removes the bran and germ, the wheat flour had only 30 percent of the minerals found in whole wheat.

Flour, lacking fiber and nutrients, is also digested far more quickly than whole grains, causing your blood sugar to spike and then drop, leading to a rise in insulin levels. You can count on more hunger and cravings, and a decrease in your ability to feel full when you're eating ground flour instead of whole grains.

So, Flour gives you minimal nutrients and spikes your blood glucose *exactly like Sugar*—truly its evil twin. As far as I'm concerned, *Flour is Sugar.* As you read along in the book, please read Sugar to be *Sugar and*

Its Evil Twin Grain Flour. But for the sake of brevity, I'll usually just call it Sugar.

I know this is hard to read—another heartbreak, like everything's being taken from you all at once. And please know there are plenty of foods left on the table for you to enjoy. Breaking up with Sugar and Flour lets you *truly* appreciate these foods. That's why I'm sharing this with you now, for the good of the beautiful long-term relationship with food that is on your horizon. Can you imagine beginning this relationship committed to your Sugar-free life, only to find yourself in the very same sad, abusive place with Flour? You know what I mean: inhaling ginormous quantities of white bread smeared with cream cheese and angel hair pasta drenched in butter, jonesing for more, more, more, feeling fat, shameful, and demoralized. There's no place for that in this big beautiful life you're creating. So while we are up and willing, let's also say good-bye to the *other* white poison.

For the love of eating

You now understand that your relationship with Sugar and Flour can be filed under "substance addiction"—like relationships with alcohol, cigarettes, and cocaine. But wait, there's more! It can also be filed under "process" or "behavioral" addiction. Like with gambling, sex, and gaming. So we have a two-for-one special of sorts. Ugh, I know. Why do I have to break this news to you? Our destructive relationship with Sugar is not only a function of its mood-altering characteristics, it also comes with its own separate lure.

Eating obviously involves way more than simply ingesting macronutrients. It includes rituals, behaviors, routines, and feelings. You know, that "hand-to-mouth" action that you find both rewarding and self-soothing in the moment. And you know how that hand-to-mouth motion very easily turns into compulsive overeating, which brings feelings of numbness, almost always followed by shame and demoralization. Without question it happens with Sugar and Flour, and it can happen with other foods as well.

Our feelings about eating—and overeating—food are often ingrained and occur quickly, without our realizing it. Reaching for the next handful of popcorn at the movies, eating the free appetizers at happy hour, or grabbing a handful of candy from your friend's desk. And there are other behaviors that are much more emotionally based— walking to the kitchen when we feel lost or bored, going to the vending machine when we're stressed or angry, or the more infamous scouring of the cabinets when we are lonely or overwhelmed at night, gorging on ice cream and cookies when we're feeling sad or scared.

Because your relationship with Sugar involves both a behavior (the act of eating) and a substance (the Sugar itself), it is hard to study brain responses solely addressing the process of overeating. What we do know is that other process addictions, such as gambling and playing *Fortnight* or *Candy Crush*, have been shown to affect your brain's motivation, reward, and impulse-control systems in the same way as substance addictions.

We can't properly address your relationship with Sugar without talking about these emotional and behavioral aspects. The fact that it's also a process addiction helps to clarify just why the feelings can get so intense and the breakup can feel so hard.

But I eat too much of everything!

Food is essential for survival. You can't say the same about cocaine, heroin, or gambling. This makes your problem of overeating very, *very* difficult; you're confronted with food every day of your life! This leads many people to be concerned about multiple trigger foods—*But Molly, I overeat cheeseburgers, nachos, pizza*; the list goes on and on. And I don't deny that, at all. What we usually see is that the foods that trigger you to obsess and binge usually contain Sugar or its evil twin, Flour. And when we narrow down your food problems to breaking up with *Sugar and Flour*, it becomes a much more manageable and solvable problem.

Why meeeeeeeee?

You may be thinking, *Thanks for the death sentence, Molly.* Ugh. *This is so unfair.* Why me? As an end-stage, full-blown Sugar and Flour addict myself, I totally get that with all my heart and soul.

It goes something like this, right? *My friend Sarah goes out to lunch with me and leaves her plate of pasta Alfredo half eaten. And then takes a few mindful bites of the chocolate mousse! Why can't I do that? This isn't fair!*

Yes, truth be told it *isn't* fair. We are all unique; our brains and bodies are different. We all come with individual vulnerabilities to binge eating, emotional sensitivity, obesity, and addiction. The answer of why *you're* in this particular predicament comes down to the programming and sensitivity of your brain, your exposure to life experiences, and your genetic predisposition.

Research can pinpoint specific genes that make you more prone to obesity and chronic binge eating. These same genes are found in people who are susceptible to developing both process and substance addictions. And these genetic vulnerabilities make you more prone to behaviors such as difficulty regulating your emotions and being more impulsive.

Our life experiences—many of them outside of our control—can also prime our brains to be vulnerable to addiction. Research shows those with post-traumatic stress disorder (PTSD) rated higher on a measure of food-addiction symptoms. Also, childhood trauma was found to be specifically linked to food addiction, binge eating, and other dysfunctional eating patterns. It should be validating to know that for those of us with trauma, our relationship with food can get very complicated.

The evidence for individual differences in your dysfunctional relationship with Sugar is overwhelming. That's for sure. But perhaps, instead of living in the "Why me?" we can move toward "That's me" and get you on the road to your solution! I, for one, have a brain that is incredibly vulnerable to addiction; I check every vulnerability box that exists. And while your vulnerabilities may be different than mine, I can tell you without hesitation that the solution is here. With this newfound knowledge, you're well on your way to a drama-free and happier relationship with food.

I Broke Up with Sugar

Margie

My life was consumed with thoughts of food: *What am I eating next? Did I eat too much? I didn't eat a lot for breakfast, so I can have more for dinner.* I woke up every morning promising myself that *today* would be a good day—*different.* And then I'd go to sleep at night hating myself because I'd binged. And every night I promised tomorrow would be better. Over and over and over again.

I did all the diets—I ate soup, fiber, grapefruit, I did Atkins. And I always lost weight and considered it a success. Until, that is, I put it all back on. And somehow the yo-yo always found me more up than down and—more destructively—still full of hateful thoughts about myself.

A friend of mine had heard Molly speak and knew of my struggles. I was always open to try anything, but when I met Molly I knew this was different. Over the next few months, I allowed her to guide me, and I put my trust in her, but I resisted somewhat. I was sure my relationship with Sugar was not as abusive as she told me it was. I told myself, *This isn't my problem. I've never heard of such a thing!* But still, I followed along. I told my husband that I was being treated for Sugar addiction even though I didn't really belong there, because it wasn't my problem. Molly helped me regulate my meals (but not in a restricting way) and cut out the Sugar and Flour. She introduced me to a food foundation that made sense and truly freed me. Although I have not been on the scale in a year and a half, it's clear that I've lost more weight than I ever have (I'm down four sizes). And unlike with all the other programs, I've actually kept it off.

But the difference doesn't stop there. It may sound hard to believe, but I am a completely different person. Happier. Better focused. *Much* more patient and loving. The noise that constantly filled my head is no longer there. I don't think about food all the time. I no longer obsess, worry, or feel consumed. My life has become much simpler. And that has allowed me to focus on the more important things in life while feeling really positive and in control. I would never have believed that breaking up with Sugar could free me in so many ways.

I Broke Up with Sugar

Jan

I was absolutely addicted to Sugar. I would pour it into everything to make it more sweet and basically lived on candy. I would cross the street without looking both ways to get a fix. I was a total junkie, and it was making my life insane and unmanageable. Like a drug, it took over my brain and made me want more of that good feeling, to great excess. I clung to Sugar for so long because I thought I needed it to self-soothe and get me through scary, unknown situations. I tried to make Sugar work for me for a *long* time and kept crashing through the floor, just one rock bottom after another.

Letting go of control is very hard. I didn't want to let other people help me. I thought I knew better than any nutritionist. I feared my body changing, or that I'd have too much or too little food. And I resented having to plan so much. I thought my whole day would be devoted to meal prep.

Now that I have broken up with Sugar, I don't fixate, obsess, or sneak around like I did before. Doing the plan is second nature, like brushing my teeth. Today I enjoy my food, and I can eat foods that would've scared me in the past. I'm so much more clearheaded. I don't feel shame around my addict-like behavior with food, and honesty gets me back after slips. I can enjoy food, but also live my life during the times when I'm not eating. My skin has cleared up and my eyes are brighter. I have realized how much Sugar and poor nutrition muted my spirit; I looked haunted. Now I am living a life that I love and look forward to each day. That is a miracle. I am happy to say that I no longer need Sugar to improve my life. If I could pass one thing on to another person, it is that if I can kick Sugar, anyone can.

Chapter 4

Defining Your Relationship:
How Bad Is It Really?
(Take the quiz. You decide.)

YOUR RELATIONSHIP HISTORY

So far, every attempt you've made to control your relationship with food has been unsuccessful.

For many years, you've tried to get a handle on it. To find some semblance of discipline, control, and freedom. Of course you didn't know, until now, that Sugar and its evil twin, Flour, were the real culprits behind your diet drama and trauma.

In order to find you the relationship of your dreams, we need to prove the case—to your mind, your heart, and even your soul—that your current relationship with Sugar and Flour is *broken*.

We're going to gather the research to make this case from a few different places. The first and most important source of evidence is *you*. If I asked about your history of managing your relationship with food and weight, what would you say? What has it looked like? Let's take a peek. I want you to write down *every* attempt that you can remember to get this issue under control, and what the outcome was—what you did, how long it lasted, how it felt during and after. This means writing down every nutritionist, doctor, cleanse, pill, quick-fix diet, and the like, its outcome, and most important, why it ended. You may be amazed at what unfolds in this exercise, so try to set aside some quiet time where you can really dig in deep.

My Relationship History

* Date
* Attempt I made to control or fix my relationship with food (diet program, cleanse, nutritionist, doctor, trainer, spa retreat, etc.)
* How long it lasted
* How I felt during the attempt
* Outcome and how I felt after
* Why it ended

HERE'S AN EXAMPLE FROM MY RELATIONSHIP HISTORY:

AGE 7: NUTRITION PROGRAM
* **How long it lasted:** 4 weeks
* **How I felt during the attempt:** Confused, like it was unhelpful
* **Outcome and how I felt after:** Ineffective. More confused than when I began.
* **Why it ended:** Program ended, didn't sign up for another session

AGE 9: WEIGHT WATCHERS
* **How long it lasted :** 2–6 weeks, on and off until age 29
* **How I felt during the attempt:** Felt hopeful each time I started the program. Convinced this would be the time. Optimistic each time they came out with a new version, then disheartened. About two weeks in I started cutting corners, not writing down food, overeating, eating foods that were off the plan, eating far more than was prescribed. I would think about ways to get around the program: not writing accurately what I was eating and hiding the food I ate, bingeing after weigh-ins.
* **Outcome and how I felt after:** Lost some weight at first, and gained it back plus more. I felt defeated and disappointed.
* **Why it ended:** I stopped attending meetings.

AGE 14: WEIGHT-LOSS SUMMER CAMP
* **How long it lasted:** 2 months per summer for 7 summers
* **How I felt during the attempt:** I felt excited at first—the idea of

dumping a bunch of weight and then showing up back at home or at college transformed was beyond exhilarating to me. In the back of my mind—and sometimes in the front of my mind—I knew this wouldn't work. Even if it was successful at first, I knew I would gain the weight I lost back again.

* **Outcome and how I felt after:** Gained all the weight back plus more each summer. Felt confused, ashamed, and hopeless.
* **Why it ended:** Program ended

If you're anything like me, you've made at least one or two attempts to take charge of this situation. But if we're being honest, it's more like thirty, three hundred, or thirty thousand. To make matters worse, some of those attempts have likely had a serious impact on your life. Perhaps you felt deprived, moody, or irritable while you did it. Maybe the attempts only lasted a day or a week. Perhaps you went to extreme lengths you never thought you would go to in an attempt to control your food and weight. Maybe you in fact *gained* weight during these attempts or gained significant weight after they failed. Again, I believe that every single time you tried, it was with the wholehearted intention of making it work for good. You believed that *this* time you would succeed. And, yet, if you're here reading with me, it's more likely that this relationship continues to plague you. You need a new plan, one with an actual solution. I've got your back.

Let's acknowledge a hard truth: If you were interviewing for a job controlling and succeeding at a relationship with Sugar, and with controlling your weight, you'd basically be unemployable. I don't say this to make you feel ashamed or embarrassed—quite the opposite; I say this to help empower you in changing course. When you can declare that you need help and that maybe you need to do this in an entirely new and different way, you allow for a whole new path to emerge.

Your best attempts—made with your utmost determination and faith—were set up for failure from the get-go. Obviously, a huge part of this problem is your relationship with Sugar. Another significant reason has nothing to do with your personality, your willpower, or even the lure of a diet. The truth about most—if not all—of your attempts is that they aren't intended for people who have relationship problems with, or addictions to food.

So up until now, you've chosen solutions that are not designed to handle your current problem with food, even though their seductive sales pitches may have tried to convince you otherwise. It's like you've been taking Advil for a serious case of strep throat—and then wondering why you can't get better—when the truth of the situation is that you've been taking something that's not appropriate for your diagnosis. You've been taking the wrong medicine: Advil is not an antibiotic. It's time to get you the remedy you need—one that helps you find freedom.

And, *of course*, you've abandoned the Sacred Vow—jumping ship, cutting and running when times get tough, instead of staying the course in your relationship! What other option is there when you're not healing? In this new life that we are creating, there's going to be a whole new strategy. The help you need is here.

WHAT'S YOUR RELATIONSHIP STATUS?

What path are you on and how harmful is it, really? How does this relationship affect *you*? That's the million-dollar question, and the only one that counts. Sadly, we don't make big, brave, sweeping, permanent changes based on general research or what happened to Emily or Sarah. This needs to be deeply personal—you need to know how Sugar affects *you* in order to be motivated to change.

Lucky for us, there's a survey designed precisely to help you better understand where your relationship stands right now. The Yale Food Addiction Scale (YFAS), developed from the diagnostic criteria for "Substance-Related and Addictive Disorders," was created by Dr. Ashley Gearhardt to assess food-addiction symptoms. It's a measure that's rooted in solid research and has been validated many times, a tool that will help you to more clearly see the current reality of your relationship. For time's sake, I've taken her survey of thirty-five questions and condensed it into twelve. If you're interested in doing the full survey, go for it! You can find the YFAS for free at https://fastlab.psych.lsa.umich .edu/yale-food-addiction-scale/.

This quiz is going to stir up a lot of feelings, especially in the form of resistance and denial. Your only job right now is to become aware of these feelings so we can move beyond them into your solution. Sugar and Flour are going to do whatever they can to convince you that none of these scenarios apply to you—and that I'm crazy, rigid, and wrong. I've sat with many of my clients while they've taken this quiz. Initially, they insist they don't relate to most of the examples. But once we are able to get the sweet whispers of Sugar out of their heads, they see that they can apply almost every example to their life and relationship. So take a deeeeeeep breath and set aside some quiet time to do this exercise. Remember, addicts naturally protect their substance. So please be mindful of whether you're inadvertently protecting yours.

I wish I were sitting right next to you while you were taking the YFAS. Since I'm not (sadly), let me remind you again: I'm not crazy, you're not crazy, this evidence-based diagnostic quiz is not crazy—but your relationship with Sugar may be. And I've been there, making every excuse in the book to protect that relationship. I'm on the other side now with so many of your people, living free of these demons—and let me tell you, it's *so* much better on this side. My freedom began with the difficult and deep acceptance of the problems that Sugar and Flour were causing in my life.

So I ask you—and maybe even beg you—to read each of these criteria slowly and conscientiously, and to take it all in. Carefully consider each of the twelve criteria and see which ones apply to you. Again, here's my sincere request: Please do your absolute best to approach each example with the most open mind and honest answer that you can possibly muster in the name of your future freedom. Pleeeeeeease?

Here we go!

☐ **1) When you eat specific foods, do you eat more than planned and past the point of hunger?**
You look at the sleeve of cookies and tell yourself you'll "just have one." Even with that conviction, you find yourself unable to stop there; you eat more than one and maybe even the whole sleeve. If you haven't committed to "just one," it's because you've resigned yourself to the idea that it's impossible.

If you've compulsively overeaten or binged before, or told yourself you'd only have a few pieces of candy and then eaten way more than that, you should check this one off.

☐ **2) Do you worry that you need to cut down on your eating, or have you tried to cut down on your eating, but found yourself unable to do it?**
You've been unsuccessful at every diet you've started. You promise yourself to start again, get back on track, or eat healthily at nine a.m., and then find yourself eating a pastry at four p.m., disappointed once again.

I think it's safe to assume that you haven't picked up this book unless you've failed at a diet or two. The cycle of telling yourself you'll "do it this time" and then ending up right back where you started (or worse off) the next hour, day, or week creates a whole host of new problems.

While this criterion is one of the hallmarks of addiction, your unsuccessful attempts to quit have reinforced the idea that you're too weak willed or lazy to make changes, and this has an impact on *all* areas of your life, self-esteem, and self-worth.

☐ **3) Do you spend a lot of time going out of your way to get food, eat food, or recover from eating food (causing you to feel sluggish or tired)?**
Going out of your way to get food: *Your favorite goodie is at a store thirty minutes away, and though you're going to be cutting it close to making it to work on time, you make sure you get your specialty doughnut before they sell out.*
Eating food: *You stay up way past your bedtime eating all of your Sugary binge foods.*
Recovering from eating: *The morning after an overeating episode or binge you wake up tired and groggy.*

The time and energy Sugar steals from us . . . whoa. When Sugar unnecessarily consumes our time and energy, we are forced to make sacrifices in other areas of our lives.

□ 4) Have you cut down or given up on doing important things in your life, as a result of your eating behaviors?

You skip your best friend's birthday party because you feel so uncomfortable and anxious at the thought of having to eat in front of others or get dressed in clothes that look good. You worry that photos might be taken of you and cringe at the idea of seeing them (or having others see them) on social media.

You call out sick for your fun-filled work event because you're worried you'll be judged for how you look or for overeating, or you'd simply rather stay home and eat.

Sugar may have prevented you from doing the things that bring you joy, like hanging out with friends or participating in your favorite activities—dancing, volleyball, that awesome Zumba class. It's also prevented you from taking risks—going for that promotion or getting back into the dating scene. You may think about life when your relationship with Sugar was more stable and wistfully remember all the things you used to enjoy doing, like meeting up for coffee, taking photos, drawing, hiking . . . the list goes on. Your relationship with Sugar doesn't allow you to spend time doing what you really want. Your time with others is overshadowed by discomfort in your body, the urge to binge, or fear that you might overeat. You have inadvertently traded some of the love of family and friends for the love of Sugar and Flour. Even if this happens some of the time and not all the time, consider checking this box.

□ 5) Have you kept eating despite emotional and physical consequences?

You're sitting across from your doctor hearing the diagnosis "insulin resistant" and learning that if your blood sugar continues to rise, you're on the fast track to type 2 diabetes. You still pick up a pint of ice cream for dessert on your way home.

You know for sure that every time you go to the Chinese buffet, you eat way too much and wake up feeling nauseated, bloated, and shameful. The next time your friends suggest a trip, you go back and repeat the same behavior.

You know eating the package of cookies comes with the risk of eating more, isolating yourself, or feeling alone and depressed, and still, you find yourself tossing the empty wrapper in the trash.

If you're in an abusive relationship with Sugar and Flour, you may have known for some time that it's hurting your health. Not only is it hurting you physically, it also packs an emotional punch. You may feel ashamed waking up each morning having broken promises to yourself. You may feel embarrassed by your body, or sad that nothing has worked. What's more, you may be concerned about the harm to your body. You may avoid doctors because you're afraid to hear about the medical consequences caused by your abuse of food. You keep going back to Sugar despite all this.

☐ 6) **Do you feel the need to eat more than you once did to feel satisfied or relieved? Do you notice that you don't get as much enjoyment from the same amount of food as you used to?**
You don't understand why all your friends can be satisfied after one cookie, one slice of cake, one piece of pizza. Those serving sizes are not helpful in your feeling full or satisfied.

When you consistently eat more and more Sugar and Flour, your dopamine and taste buds are dampened, causing you to seek out more and more. You need five sugars in your coffee instead of one. You don't consider an apple to be a sweet treat. You sadly giggle when you see the recommended serving size for pasta.

☐ 7) **When cutting down on eating problem foods, do you feel bad emotionally or physically, or have strong cravings for food?**
You stop eating Sugar for a day. You feel tired, sluggish, and irritable as you go about your life. You feel your head pound. Your thinking is foggy.

Maybe you've unknowingly started to feel these symptoms in the past and returned to Sugar to feel better in the moment. During withdrawal, you often experience a negative mood and a higher sensitivity to your emotions and overall stress. You may feel anxious or melancholy, and something deep within you is telling you the only way to feel better again is to eat.

☐8) Have you had problems with family or friends because of your eating behaviors?
People invite you out and you don't go because you feel so "fat," you're worried you won't fit in the seats, or that you'll be made fun of.
One of the main arguments you've been having with your significant other is their concern with your eating, weight gain, or the health consequences of your food behaviors.

Your relationship with Sugar pulls you deeper into isolation from others. It lowers your self-confidence, which in turn gets in the way of making and following through with plans. You may have to regularly buy new clothes, which can be expensive, shameful, and increasingly challenging the bigger you become. You often feel less-than around others. You find yourself in arguments and confrontations with concerned loved ones about these behaviors. Again, consider checking this box even if it only happens for you some of the time.

☐9) Have your eating behaviors gotten in the way of taking care of your family, fulfilling your responsibilities, or succeeding in school or work?
You're at work and become consumed by thoughts of how you're going to pick up your favorite foods for the evening—ice cream, cookies, pretzels, cake. It prevents you from finishing the task you had intended to have completed by the end of the day.
You are constantly grabbing food during your breaks and have a hard time staying focused on the work for your upcoming deadline.
You need to skip work or are late to your kids' soccer practice because of your food behavior the night before.
You secretly keep candy in your desk so you can have access to a quick fix if work gets stressful.

Thoughts of eating and overeating Sugar can be all-consuming. This can make it really hard to participate fully in work and life.

☐ **10) Have you been so preoccupied by eating or thoughts of eating that it's put you in a physically dangerous situation?**

You're craving your favorite fast food, so you get off work, make it to the drive-through, shove food into your mouth while driving, making yourself a danger to yourself and to others behind the wheel.

As a type 1 or 2 diabetic, you continue to eat sweets despite having a high blood-sugar level.

The need to indulge in your cravings can overwhelm your ability to make loving judgments, and this can impact your health and safety . . . not to mention the health and safety of those around you.

☐ **11) Have your cravings and desire for food been so strong that you couldn't think of anything else or you had to eat the foods right away?**

It's one a.m. and you have a big presentation in the morning. You're nervous, you can't sleep, and you remember the king-sized chocolate bar in your kid's backpack—5 minutes later, you've devoured it.

You go to the supermarket and pick up cupcakes for the office party. You've eaten two of them in your car, before you even made it home.

You sit home late at night craving snack food and sweets. You try hard to distract yourself with other things, but it feels impossible to think about anything else. You make multiple trips to the kitchen and pantry, and end up feeling uncomfortably full, not caring about the diet you started this week.

Cravings can be like a magnetic pull. Your behaviors follow suit—and follow the lure of Sugar—sometimes without you even realizing until it's too late!

☐ **12) Do your eating behaviors cause problems in your life or make you feel distressed?**

You keep eating Sugar and junk food despite the shame, embarrassment, and regret. You may feel your life is run by food, and you keep seeking it out even though it impacts you physically and/or emotionally.

You lie in bed, overwhelmed with shame, thinking, "How could I have done this again?"

Your body aches. All you want to be able to do is climb the stairs easily to pick up your kid at school or sit cross-legged in a yoga class.

This comes in the form of physical, mental, and psychic health distress. Oh, the food comas and Sugar hangovers. There are few things worse than waking up after a binge, or wishing you could stop eating, and failing again and again. You may feel distressed, powerless, and depressed.

THE BIG REVEAL

And now for the big reveal . . . How destructive is your relationship? How strong is Sugar's grip on your life? How many of these statements did you identify with?

You're in a relationship with:

- **2–3 statements: a deadbeat loser**
- **4–5 statements: a compulsive control freak**
- **6+ statements: a full-blown abuser**

For me, Sugar was definitely a full-blown abuser. I'm a 12 out of 12. If you're not at that level, *yay!* But sadly, that doesn't necessarily mean you ought to close this book and go out for a celebratory frozen yogurt.

Take a look at your relationship status with Sugar and consider this—do you want to have a relationship with anything in your life that's defined as a deadbeat loser or compulsive control freak? I really hope not. Even if you're not as severe as others may be, your relationship with Sugar may not be serving your health and long-term goals in food, weight, and *life*. For the love of all things *you*, you may still want to continue reading about how to break off this relationship.

There is no need to wait until you're in a relationship with a full-blown abuser to make these changes. The truth is, the sooner you nip this in the bud, the better off you will be. Here's the real and sad truth: Abuse and addiction are progressive conditions. That means they get worse over time if they're not healed. Science clearly shows that when you intervene with an addiction earlier rather than later, you have a greater chance of shortening the episode and preventing relapse. So if you agree with any of the statements in the questionnaire, it's safe to say that some change is needed. Your relationship with Sugar will deteriorate over time if you decide to stay in it without taking some positive steps in the opposite direction. I know I speak for so many in our tribe when I say I wish I had taken action earlier—it certainly would have saved me a lot of physical and emotional anguish. While it may be hard to believe it's come to this, I want you to consider a breakup, regardless of the intensity of your relationship status. Taking action is where you're freedom really lies—and you may just thank me in the end.

I Broke Up with Sugar

Christina

I came to Molly's program after a long night of eating an entire box of pasta and two boxes of cookies, and topping it off with a gallon of ice cream. Binge eating had always been a part of my life, but now at thirty-two, I felt like suddenly I was losing any type of control over my eating and, as a result, over my life. My binges were no longer manageable. I started to binge every day, going so far as to binge at work (which had previously been a safe space) and at friends' homes, even leaving social engagements because my urges to binge were so strong.

Growing up, I loved eating and came from a family who used mealtimes to connect. Very quickly, I came to associate food with shame. I was a big, tall kid, and it quickly became obvious to me that I didn't look like the other girls in elementary school. My mother, who suffered with her own struggles with weight, was constantly on a diet. When I was a child, she would buy snack packs of low-fat SnackWell's cookies to put in my lunches (I would get the diet cookies and my brother would get the Chips Ahoy!). When no one was looking, I would grab one, then two, three, four cookie packages, and suddenly I was hiding wrappers in random places all over the house. When the cookies ran out, I would eat chocolate chips out of the bakery cabinet, or take peanut butter and jelly jars to my room, eating spoonful after spoonful.

In the sixth grade, I began to diet, mimicking a friend who was also bigger. I didn't know that dieting made things worse, not better. I begged my mom to send me to "fat camp"; she said no and promised to help me make healthier choices. The bingeing continued, now with even more shame. In the eighth grade, I finally got my way and began Weight Watchers. I lost forty-five pounds. I remember it as one of the happiest—and most short-lived—times of my life.

I entered a large high school, which was very stressful, and gained weight very quickly. Eating was how I dealt with anxiety and depression, because I felt like it was the only thing I could control in my life—the thing that could make me happy quickly. Senior year, I went back to Weight Watchers and lost another forty pounds, then went to college and gained it all back, plus another fifty. I would lose weight for a period of a few months, then my willpower would crack. The more failure, the worse my eating got. I'd start eating candy bars, seemingly unable to stop. And the diet drama continued: At the end of college, I was up to 260 pounds. I had done the South Beach Diet one summer and lost eighty pounds. But then I came back that fall, and the first day out of my parents' house I ate three gigantic chocolate bars, promising myself it was a onetime thing. One time became one day and, again, I couldn't stop. The dieting went on and on—lose forty pounds and gain sixty. And so it went every year. Every slipup I had, I really felt like it was all or nothing.

When I came to Molly's program, I remember sitting with her and thinking, *Are you kidding? I can't have any Sugar ever again? You must be joking. How do you have a birthday without cake?* It was a shock to my system. But I took a leap of faith, and focused on stopping just for an hour—sometimes just five minutes. And with time, things got easier. The truth is, I was in a very abusive relationship with Sugar. When I eat it, I can't stop, so total abstinence is really beneficial for me. Giving up something that's been your best friend is hard. Eating food was my security blanket, but I realized that it was actually preventing me from living the life I wanted. I learned about what I was doing with food and why I was doing it, and that helped me tremendously. I also use skills and diversion tactics to stave off binges.

I still go out with friends and live my life. I'm most successful when I don't demand perfection for myself, but instead focus on making the best decisions I can day-to-day. I've learned how my body responds to food; I like proper mealtimes, not compromising on what I want, and taking care of myself. It's a totally different mentality than anything I've ever done. I have more power over my life and feel in control of my own body, and *that* is totally life-changing.

Chapter 5

Don't Believe Everything You Think

Chances are you're still fearful and uncertain about breaking up, even though we've gathered a whole lot of evidence to show you your relationship with Sugar is harming you. Worse than that, a security alarm has probably been set off in your brain, screaming: *Maybe it's not that bad! Maybe I just need to work out more! Maybe it's my thyroid! Maybe, maybe, maybe! How will I celebrate my birthday, my anniversary, Christmas, Thanksgiving?! I'll never have fun again! How am I supposed to go out to dinner and not eat what I want?! I need my four p.m. fix to get through the day!*

If we're going to unlock the freedom you deserve, you may want to adopt one of my favorite mottoes, ASAP: "Don't believe everything you think."

YOUR STINKIN' THINKIN'

We all have Core Beliefs that guide us through life—they've been developing since you started to think! They're formed in a whole host of ways: through what you are taught, what you are told, what you see, and what you experience. Growing up you may have seen thin, glamorous actors, business moguls, or models talking about their amazing accomplishments. This information might have led you to believe, *Thin people are happy and successful.* Or maybe you saw people in weight-loss ads saying, "I lost twenty-five pounds, in three weeks, without dieting!" and heard others around you talk about the seemingly simple ways they lost weight. Seeing and hearing this again and again may have led you to believe: *Losing weight should be easy.*

When your beliefs are repeated and reinforced—internally, by those around you, and by your life experiences—they become more and more deeply ingrained. Sometimes these beliefs are very conscious—(*Sugar comforts me*)—and you can list them as quickly as your zip code. Other thoughts are deeper down, in places we don't look that often—*I don't deserve to lose weight. It's too hard to make changes in my life.* They become so embedded in your core, you forget a time when you ever thought differently. You start to make assumptions—and judgments—based on these faulty Core Beliefs: *I'm just not someone who can lose weight. I can't live life without Sugar.*

We get into serious trouble when we don't evaluate our thoughts and beliefs as we grow and change through life, and this may be presenting a bigger obstacle than you think in creating the relationship that you deserve. One of the fundamental differences between being on a diet and being in a healthy relationship with food is a shift in your thoughts and beliefs. That's where the change begins, and that's what we are going to learn about in this chapter.

SUGAR HAS AN OWNERSHIP STAKE IN YOUR BELIEFS

Your thoughts about food, weight, and your body are impacted by the hold that Sugar has on you. These thoughts have been forming and evolving right along with your relationship with Sugar.

When relationships become harmful, like this one has, your Core Beliefs slowly and stealthily shift to rationalize and justify your continued involvement in these destructive patterns: *Everyone splurges with food. I need to eat the foods I crave. I deserve this. It's rude to not share in the cake. It's no big deal.* You probably used to feel differently, but as your relationship with Sugar has deepened and changed over time, you've begun to cling to these Core Beliefs more tightly.

Take this statement: *I cannot deal with my stress without Sugar.* When I was younger, I used to enjoy lots of activities that relieve stress:

I sang in the choir, I laughed with friends, I rode horses and snuggled with my cats. But when I was deep in my relationship with Sugar, none of those things brought me joy anymore. And the moment I felt uncomfortable about anything, Sugar was my go-to pacifier. It made me feel immediately better in the moment. I eventually realized that my Core Belief shifted from *There are lots of things I can do to relieve stress in my life* to *Sugar is the* only *thing that relieves stress in my life*. It happened in plain sight—without me even knowing!

This is where your great dilemma exists: Our thoughts are part of what drives our behaviors; we don't act without a reason. Unless we start to examine some of your dysfunctional thoughts, they will continue to interfere with and justify your harmful behaviors: buying your favorite baguettes on your way home from work because *your kids just adore French bread*. Gorging on cake at a birthday party because *what's a celebration without Sugar?* "Treating" yourself to a king-size candy bar at the movies because *the Sugar keeps you awake and focused*. You get stuck in the loop of your thoughts influencing your behaviors and then your behaviors reinforcing your thoughts. And so on and so on. You know that vicious cycle all too well.

The power struggle in your brain

You're living with two contradictory thoughts that are in a battle. You know that Sugar makes you feel good in the moment. But you also know that Sugar is harming every part of your body, mind, and spirit. What. A. Dilemma. To make matters worse, this battle is super painful for your brain, which is wired to avoid pain at all costs. In my business, we call this discomfort *cognitive dissonance*.

Because it hates discomfort so much, your brain is always looking for the quick fix to the pain game. That's why you mindlessly turn to your easier, more familiar, longer-standing belief—in this case: *Sugar makes me feel good*.

As the cycle goes on, your behaviors match those thoughts and you eat a bunch of Sugar to feel good. You instantly forget the opposing information—*Sugar is harming me*—or smother it, pushing it to the very back corner of your mind so you can have what you want in the moment. Immediacy, "easy" and familiar prevails, taking you from quick fix to hopeless shame in the blink of an eye.

That puts us in quite a quandary! In order to truly end your abusive relationship, you're going to need to come to terms with these faulty Core Beliefs and behaviors. And believe you me, those thoughts and behaviors have gotten quite comfortable sitting in the driver's seat for a really long time. The battle to let them go may not be easy . . . but we got this.

We're going to start by identifying the Core Beliefs that are blocking your way to long-term health and happiness. By creating an awareness, effectively "telling on them," we can loosen their grip and start to give you some control over their impact.

Feeling stuck? Of course you are! That's cognitive dissonance at its finest! Here are some infamous Core Beliefs to help get you started:

COMMON DAMAGING CORE BELIEFS ABOUT SUGAR, FOOD, AND WEIGHT

1. If I stop eating Sugar, I'll be boring. I won't be able to have fun anymore.
2. I won't be able to deal with stress without Sugar.
3. There are no foods to enjoy if I stop eating Sugar.
4. I need Sugar to unwind at the end of the day.
5. Cutting out Sugar will only add more stress to my life.
6. I'm just not someone who can lose weight.
7. Quitting Sugar means I can never dine out.
8. I can't have a social life without eating Sugar.
9. I need a slice of cake on my birthday.
10. I can have a few bites and be okay.
11. I'm a foodie, so I can't give up Sugar.
12. If I give up Sugar, I won't be normal.
13. I don't have time to make a big change in my life.
14. I'm too tired to think about eating healthy.
15. These cravings will never end. I will be tormented by them forever.

Now it's your turn. Take some time to really consider your Core Beliefs about your relationship with food and your breakup with Sugar. Think about the easy ones floating there on the surface and the more serious ones that lie really deep within. These might be thoughts that came up after you took the quiz in the previous chapter, reflections from a lifetime of dieting, or beliefs that you were taught as a child about food and weight. Now write them down. The list may be very long for some of you diet veterans, and in fact, the longer, the better—thoroughness gets you extra stars.

MY CORE BELIEFS ABOUT SUGAR, FOOD, AND WEIGHT

1.
2.
3.
4.
5.
6.
7.
8.
9.
10.

THE ANSWER IS NOT THE OPPOSITE; IT'S THE BALANCE

Obviously there's a part of you that knows that some of your Core Beliefs are faulty, and your faith in them prevents you from making progress in your new relationship with food and with yourself. But those thoughts have been around for just about forever, and you may be more attached to them than you realize. I'd be crazy to say, "Okay, ditch these thoughts and start thinking new ones lickety-split!" Maybe that will be the outcome when you see some of your Core Beliefs on paper (*Oh my god! I didn't realize how much that thought was sabotaging me—byeeeeeee!*). But without question, there are going to be beliefs that will not go down without a fight. And frankly, to demand their immediate surrender will only make the fight longer and harder.

For these more scheming thoughts, we're going to call on a process that cognitive behavioral therapy calls Thought Balancing. We're going to take each of your Core Beliefs and better understand its function: How does it serve you currently, and how does it support your new long-term relationship goals?

Your attachments to your feelings about food, Sugar, body, weight, and dieting can and will easily cloud your judgment, so we need to get neutral, moving toward loving. Next, you'll take a step back and think about what advice you would give someone you love struggling with this Core Belief. It's really hard to give *yourself* advice here—especially when the relationship with Sugar is still so complicated. It's ridiculously easy to fall into the trap of being biased, overly critical, and unreasonably demanding when it comes to you helping yourself. Taking yourself out of the equation may help you to fact-check and recognize the wisdom you have that you're currently unable to access.

Finally, in an attempt to establish a healthier, more functional belief—one that will lead you closer to your long-term goals—we're going to find some balance. We're going to integrate these two beliefs— the Core Belief you began with and the advice you would give to someone you love. Hopefully, this will create a truth that will work for you right now.

Buddhism refers to this balance of two extremes as the Middle Way. By finding synthesis between two competing and extreme thoughts, you take the power struggle out of the equation. You find a compromise that considers both your feelings and history with Sugar and harmonizes it with objective, true reality. More often than not, the "right now" answer lies in a less extreme view. Your Middle Way Core Belief will help to calm your brain when it feels the pain that causes it to shut down and choose the more destructive path. And with that relief, you get some needed space in your thinking pattern, allowing you to make a better, more loving choice.

THOUGHT BALANCING

Core Belief	How does this Core Belief currently serve me?	How does this Core Belief affect my new long-term relationship goals?	What advice would I give a beloved friend who believed this and was struggling like me?	Middle Way Core Belief
1. Life is boring without Sugar.	I only know how to have a good time with my friends and loved ones when I'm eating Sugar. It's what makes life feel fun!	It makes me feel hopeless, unmotivated, and scared to take risks. It keeps me away from a peaceful relationship with food.	There's so much out in the world to enjoy when you're not so focused on your relationship with Sugar.	I only know a life where I have fun with Sugar. It's scary to try new things without it. I'm willing to give it a try.
2. Cutting out Sugar will only add more stress to my life.	Sugar helps me deal with my stress. It allows me to feel safe so I don't have to make any changes.	I want a healthy long-term relationship with food—and I can't do that with my current relationhip with Sugar. *That's* stressful!	Maybe you're not looking at the whole picture. Dumping Sugar may be tough, but maybe there are benefits you don't know about—like even reducing your stress!	Breaking up with Sugar may be challenging at first, but maybe life without it would provide less stress and more peace.
3.				
4.				
5.				

Please know that when I'm urging you to create a Middle Way Core Belief, I'm not asking you to abandon everything you think—I know how invalidating that would be, especially given how deeply rooted these thoughts have become. Some thoughts are going to be more rooted than others; it's entirely understandable that you may still feel conflicted about adjusting these beliefs. Crazy as it may sound, you can realize these beliefs aren't serving you well *and* still be fearful about changing them. That's totally okay. *I'm not someone who can lose weight* can soften into *It's been hard for me to lose weight in the past, but that doesn't mean it's impossible this time.* Your beliefs can slowly shift, and with them your behaviors. And that's where the path to freedom begins.

I'm the first to acknowledge that we are pretty powerless over the ideas that pop into our heads. Still, we *do* have the power to be selective about what choose to *believe*. Don't take it too personally if you have days when your mind is full of thoughts best saved for a padded room. It's not the thought itself that's harmful; it's your belief in and commitment to it that places you further away from your overall goals. When we become more aware of what we are *thinking*, we can become more discerning about what we choose to *believe* and, essentially, the endgame: how we *behave*. And that is where all your power lies.

THE TURBOCHARGED PATH TO CHANGE: ACTION

It's certainly important to have an awareness of the thoughts that may be holding you back. Even though your thoughts influence your behavior, when you're consciously committed to an action, it can overrule any thought that you have—good or bad.

If you're someone who likes to take the fast track on getting all the things, then let me introduce you to an amazing concept of behaviorism that has helped many. Very rarely do we feel better and then act better. So while these Core Beliefs certainly have a subconscious rule in your life, the truth of behaviorism is that the money lies in *acting* your way into better thinking. If you can tolerate the noise of your sabotaging beliefs without succumbing to them, and act in this book's good faith, you can fast-track yourself to the relationship of your dreams.

Research totally agrees. Studies have shown over and over again that it's much easier and quicker to *act* your way into better habits than to *think* your way into better habits. Thinking alone is not an effective means of stopping us from doing anything—especially leaving our unhealthy relationship with Sugar. That explains why even though you've read the news articles, watched the documentaries, and heard from countless others about how Sugar is bad for your health, you still can't seem to change your behavior and ditch it for good. How many times have you thought, *I should cut down on eating Sugar. It's really bad for me*? And how many times has that helped you do . . . anything?

The truth is, making an action plan to end your relationship with Sugar—which we are going to talk about in parts two and three of this book—and then implementing that plan is the most powerful way to retrain your brain and resolve the discomfort caused by cognitive dissonance. Brain-imaging studies show us that *actions*, not thoughts, are responsible for forming new neural pathways in our brain. And those neural pathways, which are responsible for sending information from one part of the brain to another, are what control and strengthen new behaviors.

The best researched truth is that when our behaviors start changing, our thoughts almost always follow. Talk about a turbocharged path to getting where you want to go!

I Broke Up with Sugar

Michele

I've never been someone to have *one* of anything, especially when it comes to Sugar, and my relationship with food has always been tricky. I've probably done every single diet that's out there. My longest sustained diet was six weeks. Usually, I would be successful for about three weeks, then I would get angry, or some great occasion would come along, and I would say, "Of course I have to celebrate! It's not a big deal. I'll just get back on track tomorrow." But having that "one" lit up my brain for more, and the rest was downhill. That's been my experience with every single diet, including just trying to eat moderately. It didn't work for me long term. As soon as it was three or four in the afternoon, I'd be pulled to the fridge. I experienced disappointment after disappointment and felt like I could never succeed.

It never crossed my mind that I would ever break up with Sugar, because Sugar was my world. So when I first started following a meal plan without it, it was difficult. I had been so accustomed to eating whatever I wanted for as long as I wanted. I had to sweat and scream and cry for six weeks. After I got through the initial obsessions and cravings, though, it got so much easier. I now realize cravings will always pass.

I always felt like I couldn't stick to a plan for more than six weeks; breaking up with Sugar changed all that. I didn't have to struggle anymore. I could go out and do things and finally live my life. I no longer thought about food. I knew exactly what my mealtimes were, which took out the anxiety and my need to control my food. It left me with a lot more energy, and my anger subsided. Before breaking up with Sugar, I never spoke up, nor did I have my voice, self-esteem, or commitment to take care of myself. I went from hating myself to accepting myself as a person with an "allergy" to certain foods. I love myself enough to be able to do what's right for me and not care about who's around me or where I'm traveling. Self-love and self-caring were a huge core-values shift.

Now I'm not in denial about my relationship with Sugar—I know Sugar has no place in my life. I'm now educated on what happens to my body when I eat Sugar, and I recognize that it's not something I can control or moderate. I realize that the only way I can be free of my obsession with Sugar is to be broken up with it—for good. And this is about taking care of myself, not losing weight or doing a diet. I no longer believe the rationalizations, lies, and excuses like *I can't give up Sugar because I need to travel* or *I can't lose weight because my husband likes to eat out.* I now have the confidence and clarity to live my life.

Part 2

The Plan: Liberation, Not Deprivation

Chapter 6

Your 66-Day Vows

Now that you've made the decision to end it once and for all with Sugar and Flour, it's time to get started. Are you ready to create your very best relationship with food and with yourself?

Before we get started on creating your amazing new partnership, we need to talk about ground rules, your vows. Every good relationship has sincere agreements, made with integrity and honesty, to keep things moving smoothly. Creating your best life and your new relationship without Sugar is no different.

I'm going to ask you to take these vows for the next sixty-six days. To be clear, sixty-six is not a random number. Research shows that adopting a new behavior takes an average of sixty-six days to become automatic—a.k.a. a habit. And while the exact number can be different from person to person, sixty-six seems to be the sweet spot according to science.

I know what you're thinking: *Sixty-six days?! That's soooooo long!* Don't be too worried. Taking these vows doesn't mean committing to sixty-six days of perfection. Studies show that making a misstep or two when you're creating a new behavior won't impact your overall progress. But you know what does? *Reaching for Sugar on the daily.* Please, please, please keep this in mind as you read through your vows. Strive to do your best, but don't beat yourself up if slips happen—just get right back to your vows. (Confusing? I dive deeper into this concept in chapter thirteen.)

TAKING YOUR VOWS

I am going to ask you to take seven vows. They'll be the guideposts that lead you to your happy and healthy new relationship with food. When things are feeling a little cockeyed, or you find yourself hitting some potholes on the road to your new freedom, I promise you that the solution always lies in these vows:

I vow to keep an open mind.

I vow to be Sugar-*free*.

I vow to be grain-Flour-*free*.

I vow to be mindful of my volume.

I vow to eat every 3 to 4.5 hours.

I vow to be a planner.

I vow to weigh myself in a loving and accountable way.

VOW 1: I vow to keep an open mind.

Here I am preparing you for your big breakup with Sugar, and your first vow isn't even about food! That's how important having an open, flexible, and earnest mind is to your new relationship.

"You must unlearn what you have learned." —Yoda

Yoda is onto something here. Listen, I get it: You have spent days upon years upon decades in the diet drama and trauma—that struggle has been *real*. And it's left some serious scars and given you major trust issues. Like, why in the world will *this* time work? I hear you, but I need to beg you to check that belief at the door.

My clients proclaim over and over: *I know what to eat; I just don't do it.* If that's also what you're thinking, I must say that I respectfully disagree. Years of diet drama and trauma have infused your brain with conflicting C+ information, much of it in the "fad diet" category. So, perhaps you know what to eat to burn weight off, only to regain it (and more) quickly, or you know how to eat super restrictively, only to inevitably binge on ice cream and cookies. What we are going for is bigger and better than all that noise. And truth be told, if you already knew how to maintain a loving, sustainable, empowering relationship with food, you wouldn't be in this predicament.

What Yoda is trying to say is that you may think you know, but you don't know. That's some dangerous and confusing territory. It's also why we need to have a little spring cleaning, ridding your mind of all the diets of the past, all the promises, fads, and quick fixes that haven't worked for you. The clearer and more open your mind, the better, more loving, and longer-term your new relationship can be. Just like that.

"What we think we become." —Buddha

These years of diet drama and trauma have also put your confidence and self-esteem in the gutter. You've lost the thread—the real truth about who you are and what you can and can't do. Sugar has completely disempowered you. I get it: Doing something over and over— like the bingeing or promise breaking you've been participating in—can do a number on your self-esteem.

Herein lies the problem: When you're walking around spewing self-defeating, shaming lies about yourself and your experience in this world, they become a self-fulfilling prophecy. This is going to make your breakup much harder than it needs to be. Can't we make something easy for a change?

Both I and the Buddha are asking you to watch your mouth. Well, really, watch what you say *to* yourself and *about* yourself, especially when it comes to your ability to kick Sugar to the curb. As we learned in the previous chapter, the more you think something, the more you set yourself up to live it. With a history of diet trauma, your mind has surely created a slew of self-defeating and self-destructive beliefs about you and food, armed with "evidence" from all the times you've failed to stick to a diet. And we need to be mindful of the stories you tell yourself, about all the ways you've *failed* or *cheated* or *lacked will-power*, or about how *nothing ever works* so there's *no point in trying this*. These stories are simply untrue, and as your counsel, I do not advise you to sign these contracts. Watch your judgments—both of yourself and of this process. Remember, this is not a moral issue.

These judgments are manipulations by and based on a rigged game with Sugar. And the more you say them to yourself, the more power you give them to become true. So, I am asking you to keep an open mind about yourself and about this new relationship with food, to leave those stories where they belong—in the past—and to change the dialogue about what is possible for you today.

WATCH YOUR LANGUAGE: A CHEAT SHEET

* Watch (and correct) the thoughts you have in your head and the words that come out of your mouth. Both are equally toxic.
* Watch the shaming language you are using about yourself: "I'm such a: *loser, fat-ass, failure,*____ [fill in the awful blank]."
* Watch the self-fulfilling things you are saying: "I *always* fail at losing weight; I'll *never* release the weight; I'll *never* be able to give up Sugar; I *love* that peach cobbler *so much*."
* Watch the words that disempower you and make you forget you have a choice: "I *needed* to have those M&M's; I *can't* get to the grocery store today; I *need* a sweet after dinner; I *don't* eat quinoa."
* Watch the hyperbole and simple untruths—where the punishment does not fit the crime: "I'm going to *die* if I don't have that cake; It's *killing* me living without dessert; I *cheated* and had a cookie; I can't have Sugar on this *diet*." Or my very favorite: "I'm *starving*!" (Note: You will never starve to death between breakfast and lunch.)

Shoshin is a concept of Zen Buddhism, which loosely translates to "beginner's mind." It refers to having an attitude of openness and eagerness, and a lack of preconceptions when approaching a task. It's a crucial part of your new relationship, something you need in order to make this vow work. Having a beginner's mind is acting as though this is the very first time you've done this, being willing to try things as if they are entirely new to you (even if they're not), and letting go of all of your opinions, judgments, ideas, techniques, and even your beliefs.

Sometimes it will feel better in the short term to go back to your old ways. You'll find many reasons during this process to retreat and close your mind. You know what I mean: assuming things based on past experiences, being a know-it-all, worrying about not having Sugar in the future instead of focusing on the present or having a "been there, done that" mind-set. When you feel your mind shutting down, I need you to go get your pliers and pry that baby open again. And again. And again.

VOW 2: I vow to be Sugar-*free*.

Here's the biggie—and why I really need your mind wide open. You are becoming free from your abusive relationship with Sugar. Free of all the drama and despair. Free of the initial sweetness and inevitable subsequent misery.

I've broken this vow down into three categories: vowing to be free of Sugar and all its aliases, free of Sugar substitutes and artificial sweeteners, and free of drinking calories.

I vow to be *free* of Sugar and all its aliases.

Nobody knows better than you what a sneaky little bugger Sugar can be. Sugar morphs and reinvents itself (with a little help from the mad men in the food industry) into different shapes and sizes, all ready and waiting to take you down. To date, there are *at least* sixty-one different aliases Sugar hides under:

Agave, Barbados sugar, barley malt, beet sugar, brown sugar, buttered syrup, cane juice, cane sugar, caramel, carob syrup, castor sugar, coconut flakes, condensed milk, confectioner's sugar, corn syrup, corn syrup solids, craisins, dates, date sugar, dehydrated cane juice, Demerara sugar, dextran, dextrose, diastase, diastatic malt, ethyl maltol, free-flowing brown sugars, fructose, fruit juice, fruit juice concentrate, galactose, glucose, glucose solids, golden sugar, golden syrup, granulated sugar, grape sugar, high fructose corn syrup, honey, icing sugar, invert sugar, maltose, malt syrup, mannitol, maple syrup, molasses, monk fruit, muscovado, panocha, powdered sugar, raisins, raw sugar, refiner's sugar, rice syrup, sorbitol, sorghum syrup, sucrose, treacle, turbinado sugar, yellow sugar . . .

Sugar is *everywhere.* Your culprits will always be in the ingredients section—and especially in the Sugars you don't think of as Sugars: Cue the raisins, dates, craisins, coconut, dried pineapple, dried any-fruit, condensed milk, and fruit juice.

It gets worse: Sugar is so cunning, it's hiding in foods you regularly eat that you would never think to categorize as harmful. You know the obvious foods: cookies, cakes, candy, and the crew. And, yes, those guys cause major damage. But they're known offenders. It's the Sugar culprits that show up where you least expect it that you really need to keep an eye out for. It's the Sugar in your sauces—teriyaki, sweet and sour, hoisin, peanut, Worcestershire, barbecue sauce; the list goes on and on. In your dressings—French, most vinaigrettes, Thousand Island, ginger, and so many more. It's the sweetness in your condiments: sriracha, honey mustard, ketchup. Sugar finds its way into most of your packaged and processed goods—flavored yogurt, cereal, deli meats, bacon, peanut butter, and protein bars. All of this hidden Sugar can trigger hunger and overeating—even when your intentions are pure. We need to be craftier than Sugar, which means being awake and aware, knowing exactly what is in the food we're eating.

Two rules of thumb:
1. If it's too sweet to be true, it's probably Sugar.
2. When in doubt, check it out.

In our new life, we don't discriminate: *Sugar is Sugar is Sugar,* in all its shapes and sizes. Chemically, your brain can't tell the difference between organic homemade maple syrup, the packages of syrup you get at the diner, natural honey, agave, and genetically modified high fructose corn syrup. It's all Sugar, and that first bite restarts your miserable, demoralizing relationship with food.

I vow to be *free* of Sugar substitutes and artificial sweeteners.

Here's the skinny on artificial sweeteners: If it looks, tastes, and sweetens like Sugar, it's triggering the very same effect as the real deal. With the food industry's help, we've been able to convince ourselves that artificial sweeteners are "free foods," that they don't impact us at all and can even *help* in our efforts to release weight.

This is so far from true it seems like it's one of the devil's greatest coups. Artificial sweeteners are just as bad as or worse for you than Sugar. Science has proven it and your taste buds most certainly agree.

Sugar substitutes prime our taste buds to prefer sweet things. Splenda, one of the most popular artificial sweeteners, is manufactured to be an astounding six hundred times sweeter than Sugar! I know what you're saying: *But some sugar substitutes are natural! Stevia is from a leaf!* That's true, but even when it's in leaf state, it's thirty times sweeter than regular old Sugar. Once extracted, in its packaged form, it's three hundred times sweeter! Understandably, eating all these Sugar substitutes dulls our taste buds and enhances our desire for sweeter and sweeter foods. No longer is an apple—or even a coffee with one Sugar packet— satisfactory. We. Want. More. Sweet. And then we're locked in another nasty cycle.

You may be saying. "It's not *that* big a deal—I only use two sweeteners in my coffee in the morning!" You may think that's not a big deal, but it's a pretty big deal. Starting your day with something that sweet makes you crave Sugar *all day long*!

So it's safe to say that Sugar substitutes can be as triggering or even *more* triggering than Sugar itself. Research is clear that artificial sweeteners enhance your appetite, cause you to gain weight, and ultimately continue to fuel your abusive relationship with Sugar. A few studies for you to chew on:

Studies show that eating artificial sweetener raises body mass index (BMI), which measures your level of overweight. One study looked at the relationship between artificial sweetener and a change in BMI. Despite the sweeteners being calorie-free, people who consumed them doubled their risk of obesity by the end of the study, with a 47 percent increase in BMI compared to those who did not use them.

Animal studies have also helped to support this: In one study, rats who were given artificial sweetener ate and weighed more compared with rats who ate Sugar. Researchers believe artificial sweeteners may interfere with our natural physiological processes by tricking our brain into thinking we need more Sugar. Because our brain registers a sweet taste with fake Sugar but our body doesn't have calories to consume, our body gets confused and isn't able to do its job properly. Research shows that artificial sweeteners enhance appetite and hunger—because, Helllooooo! Where are the calories? This causes you to overeat.

If impacting your appetite and weight isn't enough, studies show that consuming fake Sugar impacts how your body responds to Sugar itself. Artificial sweetener affects your glycemic and insulin responses, which makes your body worse at processing Sugar. What's more, sweeteners have been found to change gut bacteria, causing glucose intolerance.

Artificial sweeteners endlessly feed your Sugar cravings and abusive relationship keeping the attachment front and center in your heart and mind. My most successful clients are brave enough to completely give up their artificial sweetener habits and report *almost no cravings* for Sugar. They're the ones with the most freedom—physically, mentally, and emotionally.

I vow to be *free* of drinking my calories.

Sugar also lurks in a bunch of drinks you might not think have any at all—adding extra calories and extra Sugar—making you hungrier when you consume them.

Drinking your calories in the form of any juice—even organic fresh pressed—is mainlining Sugar. Without the fiber of fruit and veggies in their whole form to slow the Sugars down, you're basically drinking juice-heroin. The speed with which the liquid hits your endocrine system is far more than it can handle, spiking your insulin, crashing your blood sugar, and dulling your dopamine receptors. And that's the same for all drinks that have calories.

So scratch the health benefits of juice cleanses, kombucha, coconut water, Gatorade, electrolyte mix, green juice, organic celery juice, and *any* juice. And scratch the health benefits and convenience of drinking smoothies. Same deal—drinking your calories lands you back in your abusive relationship with Sugar, which is of no health benefit. *At. All.*

The science is clear that drinking your calories keeps you unknowingly in a destructive cycle with Sugar: There is a bunch of data that indicates chewing allows for feeling full, while *not* chewing makes you more hungry. Suzanne Higgs, a professor at the University of Birmingham, studies the psychobiology of appetite. She found that students who chewed their lunch for longer had less snacking later in the day, which suggests that chewing can impact your feeling full after a meal. Other research has found that chewing may have an effect on the feeling we get when we've had enough to eat. Several studies have found that chewing more can reduce food intake, lower hunger, and increase fullness.

Drinking our calories is more than our insulin receptors can handle. Sugar in its liquid form enters our bloodstream at such a fast rate that our pancreas is alerted to produce more insulin than needed. Extra insulin causes hunger and cues your body to store fat—both things that we have absolutely no interest in, and that take us further from finding our dream relationship.

My favorite study comparing eating apples to drinking apple juice shows that drinking your calories makes you more prone to blood sugar crashes, which causes fatigue and cravings—both things that you want to avoid in your new beautiful life.

So the data on this is clear: Drinking your calories keeps you entangled in your unhealthy relationship with food and works against your weight-release goals. If you're wholly resistant or unwilling to give it up, your relationship with juice and smoothies may be more codependent than nurturing.

A quick note on your favorite way to drink your calories: alcohol.
Before you start rationalizing boozing it up, let me just say: Happy

hour can be happy, and sometimes it can be really messy and not so happy. Simply put, *your resolve dissolves in alcohol*. After a couple of cocktails, that nacho plate on the bar calls your name. You go from "Heck no" to "Plate of mozzarella sticks, please" without even realizing it.

While I would love for you to be free of Sugar *and* alcohol, I know that isn't a realistic life for most people. So when it comes to drinking, I'm asking you to look at quantity and quality. While zero booze is ideal, we suggest maxing your alcohol intake to two servings per week. And as your friend, coach, and trusted part of your Power Circle (more on this in chapter sixteen), I say this with deep love: If two cocktails a week doesn't seem like a limitation that you can handle, you may want to take a closer look at your relationship with alcohol.

A serving of alcohol is one ounce of hard liquor in my book. Be sure that the booze you choose is Sugar-free. Gin, vodka, and whiskey are the dry alcohols with the lowest fructose levels. These can be mixed with a noncaloric liquid like seltzer. And let's be sure to leave alcohol in a category of its own. No robbing Peter to pay Paul here—if you're having a drink, it's an addition to, not a substitute for, any part of your meal plan. Vodka soda is not a snack. Or a meal.

We also need a little fact checking here: Alcohol *is* Sugar. Which means it lights up our brain the same way Sugar does. As a result, there are many people in the "full-blown abuser" relationship status who find it extremely difficult to stay away from misusing Sugar and Flour when alcohol is involved. It's not that they're alcoholics per se, but they're Sugar addicts who can't drink without bingeing.

VOW 3: I vow to be grain-Flour-*free*.

As I said before, Flour is Sugar's brother from another mother. As it turns out, your body and mind have the same reaction to grain Flour as they do to Sugar. And if you really think about it, this should resonate for you. Pizza, which I can eat endlessly, is a whole lot less exciting without the doughy crust. Hot dogs can be a summer treat, but pigs in the blanket, or a hot dog on a warm, toasted potato bun makes my mouth water.

Just to be clear, I'm not asking you to vow to be free of *grains*, just free of the Flours manufactured from them. Why? In chapter three, we learned that when you eat Flour, your body reacts to it as if it is Sugar, causing quick blood-sugar and insulin spikes. That's why Flour—especially in the form of starch and most commonly found in modified food starch, potato starch, tapioca starch, and cornstarch—is just as bad as its sneaky evil twin, Sugar.

And Flour, just like Sugar, is hiding in almost *everything* you are eating. It's thickening your sauces, gravies, and soups and adding texture to your chips, fries, and puffs. We need to outsmart Flour by being vigilant about checking the ingredients in everything we're eating.

Like Sugar, the two rules of thumb apply here, too:
1. If the food's too textured and thick to be true, it probably has Flour.
2. When in doubt, check it out (the ingredient list, that is).

Are there some Flours that get a stamp of approval? It depends. Some people can handle almond or chickpea Flour, while others find that adding the less common non-grain Flours triggers their hunger response, leaving them wanting more. You decide: If you're waking up in the middle of the night bathed in cassava Flour, I suggest you put that on your red-light list immediately.

VOW 4: I vow to be mindful of my volume.
As the old adage goes, there is no free lunch. Cue audible sigh. It's awful—I agree. And yet if you want this new relationship with food to work and really serve you, you're going to have to accept that volume matters. A lot.

Which means you're going to need to be mindful of how much you're eating. I've watched clients kick Sugar to the curb only to find themselves in a relationship with volume that looks a whole lot like their relationship with Sugar. They experience weight gain and feel groggy, hopeless, angry, and depressed—all Sugar- and Flour-free! If you're going to gain weight and be miserable, shouldn't it be from something exciting, like bagels, pizza, cake, and candy instead of Brie, brown rice, peanut butter, and oatmeal?

For so many of us, eating large volumes of food is habitual, soothing, and comforting: *I deserve it. It's only a little more. I just need to numb out.* We need to retrain your brain and undo these antiquated habits that are getting in the way of your happiness.

What's the most accurate and effective method to manage the amount of food you consume? Weighing and measuring your food. At least in the first sixty-six days of your breakup, until your awareness is reawakened and your eyes heal.

The truth of the matter is, environmental factors and triggers cause us to overestimate what we need and underestimate exactly how much we're eating. You might have heard of this concept as "mindless eating."

Of course, we all wish that we could rely on our intuition—our internal cues—to tell us when to stop eating. What a dream! Sadly, studies show that restrained eaters (a.k.a. dieters) and people with higher BMIs don't have very good natural stop valves. External cues like a TV in the background, supersized containers, and large portion sizes tend to prompt people to keep eating rather than promote feelings of being full and satisfied.

When it comes to day-to-day decisions about food, we tend to underestimate the number of food-related decisions we make and the impact our surroundings have on us. The more distracted we are by them, the more mindlessly we eat. What a dilemma!

The solution? Weighing your food. By weighing out exact portions, you can completely avoid these traps. I'm not asking you to *like* weighing and measuring your food, or to be excited and jubilant while doing it. I am simply suggesting—strongly—that it's a good idea, one that has stood the test of time and will help you get a grip on your volume dilemma. Consider it with all of your beginner's mind—at least in your first sixty-six days, whenever you are able—while you are establishing the foundations of your new relationship.

Remember, some effort is always better than no effort. So while I would love for you to buy a travel scale and bring it with you on all your life adventures, if you're not willing to do that, please focus on how much you're truly eating whenever you can. Remembering that your eyeballs are a very unreliable source of accurate information!

Weighing your food prevents you from undereating and overeating. It also ensures that you will get everything in the right amount at every meal and every snack. When you're unsure of your portions, it's like eating your meals with a blindfold—and that's not fair to your brain *or* your stomach. Remember, knowledge is power.

For right now, as we begin delving into your new relationship, take this vow to weigh and measure your food and see what happens. Pleeeeeease? Maybe it won't be as awful as you think! Maybe you will love the freedom from not constantly having a battle in your head. That may sound counterintuitive, but you know what I'm talking about: *Maybe I should have a little more. Maybe this isn't enough. Maybe I will be hungry later if I don't eat it all. Maybe I will be too full if I eat all that.* Weighing the food stops all that noise—and that's some serious freedom.

Will I have to measure food for the rest of my life? First of all, the rest of your life is a *really* long time. But you probably won't. Your eyes can adjust to your new portion sizes and you will learn what works for you and what doesn't. You may want to measure some of the higher-calorie foods like nuts and cheese—I almost always do, just to be on the safe side. And from time to time, if your weight release plateaus or spikes a bit, you may find it helpful to return to and honor this vow in its truest form.

VOW 5: I vow to eat every 3 to 4.5 hours.
Some of you eat like chipmunks, grazing and eating little snacks here and there all throughout the day. Some of you eat like camels, gorging on one big meal that makes you so full—and probably so nauseated— that you're in no state to eat after. Some of you are a little bit of both. None of you are eating in a safe and sustainable way, which is one of the biggest roadblocks to your success. One of the most important vows

you can take is to get consistent with your eating times. The *when* to eat is just as important as the *what* to eat.

Virtually all the data on successfully overcoming binge eating reinforces this very point. Research tell us that people who struggle with their weight snack frequently, eat large portions, binge-eat, and miss meals. Sound familiar? Also eating fewer than three times a day is tied to a greater risk of weight gain and type 2 diabetes. And that's not just a weird coincidence. Skipping and restricting meals can put your body into "starvation mode." When this happens, your taste receptors have an increased sensitivity to sweet taste. So while you may *think* eating less frequently helps you lose weight, you're actually putting yourself in a more vulnerable position to eventually overeat or binge. Waiting too long between meals can cause your blood-sugar levels to dip, making you Level 11 emergency hungry. And rabid hunger makes it nearly impossible to make decisions that support your new relationship.

Research tells us that the timing of your meals is essential. It's crystal clear that skipping meals and waiting too long to eat, both habits that have likely come into your relationship, make you more likely to turn to Sugar and make it more difficult to control your body weight.

The truth is, your eating behaviors and hunger cues have run wild. Which means you'll need to go through some serious retraining of what it really means to be hungry and to be full. That's what makes this vow so important—it structures your eating so you can have the freedom of having a big beautiful life between meals and snacks. And if you're someone who says *What's a mealtime?* or *I eat when I feel like it!* Fear not. Making set times for when to eat (along with how much) will help you recalibrate your sense of hunger and fullness. Research shows that our body can totally learn hunger with some consistent timing of meals. So if you're thinking "I could never be hungry for breakfast," think again. With appropriate portions and consistent meals, you're less likely to overeat and on the road to re-training your body to know when to eat and when to stop eating.

In taking this vow, I ask you to do your best to not let more than 4.5 hours go by between any meal or snack. The 3- to 4.5-hour guideline ensures that you are protected from any urges to binge, restrict, over-eat, or under-eat. Trust me when I say it's soooo much easier to avoid that seductive and opportunistic Sugar when you are fed, feeling satis-fied, and knowing when your next meal is coming.

VOW 6: I vow to be a planner.
It's like they say in the Marines: "Fail to plan, plan to fail." Creating your new relationship with food has very little to do with willpower (as we learned in chapter three) and almost everything to do with plan-ning. Research tells us that when you approach a tricky situation with a plan, you end up following through with far more consistency than tackling the situation with the all too common "Eh, I'll just figure it out when I get there" mind-set. Because you *know* how often we actually figure it out when we get there. Basically never.

What do I mean by becoming a planner? I mean planning in every shape and form you can think of. More planning equals *better*, at least in the first sixty-six days of your breakup. The more structure you can weave into your life, the easier you make it for your brain to adapt to this new life—and the better your chances of creating lasting love in your relationship with food.

I want you to plan what you are eating, when you are eating, your meals when you dine out, and your snacks and meals when you're on the go. Think ahead to when you're going to the grocery store and ex-actly what you're going to buy there, plan your online orders, plan when you're going to prepare your food for the week, and plan when you're going to plan your planning.

As a study about exercise and planning showed, participants who set goals and planned when, where, and how to exercise vastly im-proved the likelihood of achieving their goals. Of course, this is also the case with planning with food: Meal planning is associated with eating a healthier diet and having lower body weight.

Despise planning? That's okay. You don't have to love or even like it in order to do it. My suspicion is that it will actually grow on you. I'm serious! I've seen it give a feeling of comfort and security to so many of the people I've treated—not to mention myself! Knowing what's ahead of you with a little planning makes life, with all its twists and turns, exponentially easier to deal with.

And remember, *you won't need to plan at this level of intensity for the rest of your life*. Every big change requires great effort at the beginning, because you are still learning and healing. Trust me, soon enough you'll be so deeply engaged in your beautiful life, you won't even realize that planning is your second nature!

VOW 7: I vow to weigh myself in a loving and accountable way.

It's been my experience that when you get on a scale to check your progress you become like a Vegas gambler—willing to sell your soul for just a little more. I've seen people act in the *craziest* ways around the scale. I've seen them binge after, get naked in front of me, miss time at work to recheck their weight after meals, spend thousands of dollars on multiple high-end scales, and obsess for days and days. The truth of the situation is: Weight release is an outcome, not a goal. I'm not saying it isn't important—and even essential—for your physical and emotional health. I'm simply saying that being hyper-focused on your weight has not helped you to get closer to releasing it. We need to find a better way.

There is data that says that daily weigh-ins can help release weight and keep it off. Even though research says that weighing regularly helps to release weight, it's also true that weighing too frequently is linked to unhealthy behaviors, like bingeing or restricting your food. Weighing yourself too much also has been shown to have negative consequences on self-esteem, depression, and anxiety.

So, while weighing yourself can be an important tool in releasing weight, spending too much time with the scale can have serious repercussions when it comes to your weight and body image, taking you far, far away from your loving, happy new relationship.

Where does that leave you and your scale? One size does not fit all in this vow—so you need to figure out the best method for you that will help you stay accountable to releasing weight without triggering any of the screwball scale behavior that I've described. Make a hard decision to weigh yourself at predetermined times, either twice monthly (on the first and fifteenth of the month) or monthly (on the first of the month), and don't deviate from this schedule—especially if you're "feeling" thin or fat. The point of this vow is not to determine your value from a number on a scale, but to ensure that you're moving in a direction toward optimal physical health.

In that vein, and because scales can be kooky, keep your factors consistent: weigh undressed, in the same place, at the same time, on the same scale, before you've put anything into your body.

You are looking to rid yourself of the judgmental, obsessive, shameful thinking that comes with weighing yourself, and this weigh-in commitment finds a balance between obsessing about your weight release and ignoring it completely—two patterns I see way too often.

Remember, you want to be free from your abusive relationship with Sugar and Flour, and your infatuation with the scale can turn on you in the very same way your relationship has—defining your worth, making you act out in ways that are incredibly harmful to your long-term goals, and stealing from you by making you obsess over a simple number. No. More. Drama.

Please do not read this and think that I am cool with you not releasing weight. If you are in an unhealthy weight range and are pursuing this new relationship with food with the integrity and respect that I've suggested, you will release weight. The scale is simply a reinforcement that you are moving in the right direction, *not a definition of your worth*.

These vows may be a tad intimidating, but they are totally achievable. You've got this. And with your open mind (vow one!), you'll be on the road to love, honor, obey in your long-term, loving relationship before you even know it!

I Broke Up with Sugar

Heather

My disordered eating began at a very early age. Dieting began shortly thereafter and would continue for a long time. It would always begin well, with hope and a belief that this time would be different, this time I would finally have the willpower to succeed. Sooner or later, I would crash and burn. People who loved me would say, "You just need to want it bad enough," or "When you are ready to do it, you will." Those words became weapons I attacked myself with. I always—repeat, *always*—believed that I was a failure for not having the strength to stop overeating.

I was a dancer from the time I was three, and my head instructor was a mentally abusive woman obsessed with weight. At age eight, I began to throw up after I ate. I was bulimic until I was sixteen. That was the first time I entered therapy for an eating disorder. My struggle with bulimia continued on and off throughout college. Finally, I was able to cease throwing up, but compulsive overeating would follow me for the next twenty years, until I arrived at Molly's door at age forty.

Sitting in Molly's office for my assessment, I cycled through a surprising range of emotions. I had walked in without much hope, but was desperate to be proven wrong. To say my previous attempts at gaining control over food had left me jaded would be an understatement. I had hesitantly walked through her door and braced myself on her couch, desperate for an answer. Not that I hadn't searched for one elsewhere. I had the self-loathing born of an endless string of failures. Even so, no one really got it. No one's story ever closely mirrored mine until that day.

When I met Molly, it was a surprising series of "me toos!" I was floored. That day in her office, I learned that I was, and am, a food addict. It was hard to hear, but it felt so right that I couldn't stop smiling. Molly was thrilled I was there—she sincerely believed she could help free me from this endless cycle. A small flame of hope was lit, and I was scared. Would I fail again? Would I succeed? In that moment, I am not sure which was a scarier prospect for me. My identity was rooted in the belief that I was too weak to be healthy. Sure, I could be thin, but I could never sustain a healthy weight without having an eating disorder or white-knuckling a diet to exhaustion. Break up with Flour and Sugar? Adherence to this would allow me to live freely? I was skeptical, but I was all in.

The first six weeks were difficult. The shame, fear, and self-hatred that went along with my night bingeing inspired me to persist. I did not want to go back.

And so it went, each stage easier than the previous but challenging in its own way. One foot in front of the other until my fear of going back was eventually dulled by the momentum of moving forward. I am writing this with nearly a year of adherence to Molly's program. I fully expect to be doing this for the rest of my life—I embrace it. This is why: I no longer obsess about food all the time. No longer are cravings in control, with me along for the ride. It's been a lifelong war with myself that I thought was destined to continue. There is room in my heart and mind for more now, and I love that.

The truth is that diets do not work for addicts. Who would set an alcoholic adrift in a sea of cocktails and blame their willpower if they fell in? After breaking up with Sugar, my life has gone from black and white to Technicolor. So on I will go, one day at a time, learning to see myself in this different light. Until Sugar was out of my life, I could not begin a healthy relationship with food. It was not about my willpower. It was about my understanding and acceptance of who I am and what I need.

I Broke Up with Sugar

Paul

Breaking up with Sugar changed my life. I have struggled with my weight since childhood. Over the years, I saw numerous nutritionists and dietitians and read the latest fad-diet books in a never-ending struggle to lose weight. In each case I successfully lost weight, only to gain it back plus more. It was a roller coaster.

Then I met Molly. I decided to work with her, and I am so fortunate that I did. She taught me to be mindful of the why, when, and how as it relates to eating, not just the what to eat. Most important, she told me something that none of the other nutritionists or dietitians ever did: Flour and Sugar are unhealthy and addictive.

With Molly's guidance and coaching, it was not difficult to break up with Flour and Sugar and to change my relationship with food. I wasn't put on an unsustainable diet like the other times I'd tried to lose weight. To the contrary, I completely changed my behavior toward food. Now I'm happy to say I've lost weight without being on a diet! I have made a lifestyle change in the way I eat and as a result I am thinner, happier, and healthier, and I feel much better about myself.

Chapter 7

Your Food Plan: It's Not About the Food. And It's All About the Food.

What's a new relationship with food without . . . the food? We're going to make this one stronger and better than any relationship you've had. You're going to feel secure and committed—no longer afraid of the havoc wreaked by Sugar and Flour and the inevitable pain that follows.

You're going to feel full and satisfied, while still releasing your weight. You'll no longer be a victim of starvation or a hostage to fad diets and Sugar, and you'll have a plan of eating that you can easily follow day in and day out. You won't believe the stability, confidence, and serenity that will unfold.

You may be thinking right now that breaking up with Sugar is a death sentence. Chill. You're just in the part of the breakup where you think you'll never love anything like Sugar again. That couldn't be farther from the truth. First of all, breaking up with Sugar allows your brain and your taste buds to have a whole new experience of food. When you've gotten untangled from the hijacking of your brain, food will simply taste better. But there's more—as it turns out, there is a host of foods you're going to introduce into your life that are colorful, delicious and exciting—who would have thought you could make asparagus noodles with pesto? Or wrap a cheeseburger in a collard green and eat it guilt-free? The point is your options are abundant (thanks, internet!); you're just in the middle of a breakup. I promise that you will find great love in the foods that you will choose to eat—and this time they will love you back.

If you've read ahead and snuck a peek at the Relationship Rebuild Plan (RRP), your diet radar may be screaming, "Code red!" You may be thinking, *Hold up. This "plan" feels a whole lot like another restrictive diet!* I hear you, and you're only *sort of* right.

The time you've spent eating compulsively, heavily restricting, yo-yo dieting, and being a slave to Sugar has completely demolished your food foundation. We need a serious intervention to get rid of the debris and put you back on solid ground. Your RRP is designed to help you escape the abusive Sugar cycle you know all too well. If you can imagine it, you're going to gain the ability to experience authentic hunger and fullness, so you're not left constantly wanting more. It's one of the hidden benefits of all this—a brand-new outlook and understanding of food.

While I was still in the throes of my abusive relationship with Sugar, more was more and bigger was better—it was the name of the game. I needed the largest portion possible, and even that never felt like enough. Grande or venti latte with vanilla syrup? Venti, of course. I remember going out for Italian dinners with friends and watching with utter envy as they ate half of their pasta and casually left the rest. If more food was there, I ate it, no questions asked. There wasn't a bowl big enough to satisfy me. A snack bag or value-size bag of pretzels? Value size—now! Snack-size bags just left me angry and looking for more. So you can imagine my surprise and amazement when I broke up with Sugar and found that I felt truly satisfied by my nuts-and-apple snack, or when I took the vanilla syrup out of my latte and didn't miss it. And I've treated thousands of clients who feel the same way. Sometimes my meals are so fulfilling, I actually leave food on the plate! I know, right?! Ten years later and I can still hardly believe it.

Rebuilding your foundation may feel a whole lot like a restrictive diet, but only at first. I promise. I'd like us to think of it as a reframe. It's a new way of thinking about this problem to get on the path toward a solution, ASAP. *Your RRP is not restrictive; it's protective.* We've agreed that the way you manage your food is, well, unmanageable. You need a structured and protective prescription. Without the RRP "life preserver" providing a stopgap and keeping you afloat, you're still on the same unstable ground, making you super vulnerable to more diet drama and trauma. And ain't nobody got time for that.

Your 66-day food plan is a complete reconstruction of your food foundation—the building blocks of your new relationship with food. The ultimate goal is for you to create a meal plan that works best for your own recovery—so that it meets all of your emotional, relational, and behavioral needs. I've worked with my friend and superstar nutritionist, Nikki Glantz, to ensure that it's also healthy, sound, and nourishing. It's your starting point and it's also your reset button, the place to which you can return should you ever find yourself falling off track.

I'm going to go through your Relationship Rebuild Plan step-by-step, walking you through the ins and outs, teaching you why and how the plan was created, and addressing all the questions you'll likely have in between. Unlike with every single diet you started and stopped and that inevitably failed you, I am committed to helping you be in control and feel empowered in your new life. And for the times when that's simply too hard, I've devoted chapter thirteen to what you should do when you don't want to do what you know you're supposed to do. Suffice it to say there is a lot to learn.

Your Relationship Rebuild Plan addresses the big questions when it comes to your food: WHAT, HOW MUCH, and WHEN you eat. Let your Relationship Rebuild Plan begin!

WHAT AM I EATING?

Your food plan consists of five major food groups: protein, carbohydrates, fat, fruit, and vegetables. I know you think that kicking Sugar and Flour to the curb is a great punishment, but it's very much a gift. I don't expect you to feel that way today, but know that with time, this new relationship will be paying you back, rather than robbing you.

Like all new relationships, this one will have a bit of a learning curve. And learning to live without Sugar and Flour may take the prize for most challenging. Be patient, be kind, and be tolerant with yourself— you'll be mastering the food before you know it, I promise.

Absolutely *no* Sugar and Flour?

If you haven't learned this by now, I'm a realist. I abide wholeheartedly by Voltaire's adage: "Perfect is the enemy of the good." Every meal for the rest of your life is definitely not going to have *zero* traces of sugar in it— because that's not a sales pitch for a big beautiful life, is it? And yet, when we let our boundaries get too flimsy around Sugar and Flour, they sneakily come back into our lives faster than we can say "cupcake." And I don't know about you, but I can say "cupcake" pretty darn fast.

So while I want you to try, rather perfectly, to eat foods that don't contain Sugar or Flour, we need to have a guideline that defends against your breakup becoming a makeup. Welcome the *Fifth-Ingredient Rule*: If Sugar or one of its plentiful aliases or Flour are listed as the fifth ingredient or later, that food has the green light.

Here's the step-by-step: Ingredients in packaged foods are always listed in descending order. First come the ingredients that are present in the highest quantities, and then gradually down to the ingredients with the lowest quantities. Every product has a nutrition label. Find it. At the very bottom you will find the ingredients. Read the first four ingredients. If Sugar, Flour, or any of the words that mean Sugar and Flour—words that end in -*ose* (glucose, dextrose, fructose, etc.) or *starch*—are listed in the first four ingredients, you do *not* eat that food. Again: **If Sugar or Flour are listed as the fifth ingredient or later, the food is good to go!**

Side note: You'll want to head back to your second Vow in the previous chapter to brush up on the sneaky aliases. I promise you, ignoring them puts you at high risk for an accidental run-in with your abusive relationship, leading you to overeat and experience hard-core cravings when your intentions are pure. No need to throw unnecessary wrenches in the plan! With careful attention to the Fifth-Ingredient Rule, outsmarting that sneaky sucker Sugar is easy.

All the foods (except for the real *jerks*)

This food plan is about liberation, not deprivation. I want you to be eating delicious foods you love and that love you back. As you're reviewing the plan, it may take you back to your diet-drama-and-trauma days. I'm suggesting some old-school classics like yogurt, Wasa crackers, canned tuna, Laughing Cow cheese, and more. And I'm psyched to do it.

In your new relationship, I want to put every single food that has ever been created—without Sugar and Flour—back on the table. It's in the best interest of your new relationship to have all the foods that can help build your best life available, so you can really get a sense of what you want this new relationship with food to look like.

Eating cottage cheese, should you choose to, may make you feel like you've gone back to your diet from the 1980s. But as I've mentioned before, after some time without Sugar and Flour, your brain will naturally reset and your perspective will shift. So who knows what you'll like? A couple of weeks from now, you may be enamored with cottage cheese. I know. Let me tell you, cottage cheese now rocks my world—it's *beyond* delicious on a slice of Ezekiel brand sprouted whole grain bread, in the mornings, or as an afternoon snack with some fruit and cinnamon.

So many of us are traumatized by old-school diet foods—trust me, I get it. But when I give you the game plan for your new life, I want everything to be an option for you to take or leave, even if it's cottage cheese.

Isn't fat the problem?

Remember the 1980s and '90s, when we were voraciously eating honey mustard pretzels and fat-free muffins with reckless abandon? Me too. Sigh. Fat got such a bad rap, but soon you'll understand that it isn't the enemy—it's your secret ally.

Poor fat! It was the villainized victim of such a smear campaign for so many years! Even I spent a majority of my career being taught and teaching others that fat was the problem. Don't get me started about the Sugar industry paying Harvard scientists in the 1960s to blame fat for heart disease. . . . Another story for another time. The point is, we've been led astray. Not just a little astray, but *really* astray. Our friend research tells us that fat affects our body much differently than Sugar.

While Sugar cues our brain to keep eating and not feel the effects of fullness, fat actually sends the proper "stop" message to the brain.

But be mindful. There are two ways that fat can become your foe rather than your friend. First, if you're engaging with processed foods that are bliss-point-designed—with high fat *and* high Sugar, which is a state that nature never intended—you may feel fat is a trigger food for you. Luckily, removing Sugar and Flour from the menu solves this predicament. Your other heads-up is the caloric density of fat. Fat holds a lot of calories in pretty small portions—so if weight release is part of your motive, be mindful of your fat portions. It's why one study found fat overconsumption to be linked to being overweight, even though Sugar was identified as the culprit in addictive eating.

Not all carbs are created equal

When I tell people that I've broken up with Sugar and Flour, they immediately assume that I don't eat carbs. First and foremost, that is not a life worth living, nor is it a sustainable or enjoyable relationship. And I've promised you both those things from the get-go.

Remember this: Not all carbs are created equal. Carbohydrates are an important part of every meal plan. They give you energy, and frankly, they're delicious. So it's not about *no* carbs—it's about *slow* carbs. We know from a multitude of human and animal studies that carbs—fruit, vegetables, nuts, and whole grains—are digested and absorbed more slowly, so they keep you satisfied longer, and they increase fat oxidation, which promotes weight release. This is especially true if you're insulin resistant—which applies to most of us diet veterans. And eating a diet of quickly digested *fast* carbs, like Flour, cereal, or processed snack foods, makes an insulin-resistant person more prone to develop type 2 diabetes. And we're most definitely going to avoid that.

Something to keep on your radar: I've seen how some RRP-friendly carbs such as oatmeal, brown rice, and Ezekiel bread can be trickier for some people to eat in, how shall I say it, a "respectful" way. If you're falling under this umbrella, you may choose to have these carbs more sparingly (or not at all). The RRP gives you a lot of leeway in deciding which carbs work best for you—you're calling the shots. Breaking up with Sugar means that you've freed yourself from the carbohydrates that hold you hostage and steal your thunder—be sure the carbs you're eating are helping you to feel liberated.

What about fruit?

The second question people ask about my breakup is, "What about fruit?" Fruit is natural, nutritious, and delicious, which are all components of your big beautiful life. It is true that fruit is made of fructose—which is by definition Sugar. But, most often, fruit doesn't impact your blood sugar in the same way that brownies and ice cream do. That can be attributed to one of our BFFs, fiber. Fruit is rich in fiber, and fiber helps to slow the absorption of Sugar into your bloodstream, which chills out your insulin levels and helps you avoid blood-sugar spikes.

Side note: Some fruits, such as bananas, grapes, and pineapple, can be a bit tricky, as they have higher concentrations of Sugar, which may cue some serious cravings if you're insulin resistant or have a "full-blown abuser" relationship status (as I know from the research and my personal relationship with mangoes). You decide what fruits work for you. You're the boss, applesauce!

There's a lid for every pot

Have you ever sat at brunch with people who are on different food journeys? The choices, questions, and opinions abound! Does this have gluten? Can you make my omelet without oil? Can you make my omelet with extra cheese? Can I have a salad instead of the toast? (Okay, that one is me.) Do you have any almond milk? Is there a vegan option? Are the eggs cage-free? Can you use a Sugar-free dressing on the salad instead of the French dressing that is offered? (Okay, that one is me, too.) You get the idea.

As my mom would say when talking relationships, "There's a lid for every pot." We're each on an individual journey when it comes to our relationship with food; the restrictions, allergies, ideologies, and preferences we hold make the journey unique. The RRP supports your personal path wholeheartedly. It's full of options for people who want and need them: vegan, vegetarian, dairy-free, gluten-free, pescatarian, vegan, nut-free, soy-free, love cheese, hate the texture of yogurt—the list goes on and on. The point is, everyone can participate in the RRP, on their own terms.

Side note: You may be worried about taking Sugar and Flour out of the equation if you're already subscribing to a lifestyle that eliminates foods. In my experience, people whose primary focus is the elimination of Sugar and Flour have gained more freedom than they knew was possible. I've had clients who start the RRP dairy-free and then add back some cheese in their salads and milk in their coffee while they're kicking Sugar to the curb. It resulted in their feeling freer and healthier than ever. I've had clients who had chosen a vegan lifestyle temporarily add some eggs and salmon and experience real liberation from their abusive relationship with food. Sugar and Flour are the *real* offenders. You may want to make a few adjustments—even if it's just in the beginning of your journey—to let the impact of a Sugar- and Flour-free life really take hold.

If you have a nut allergy, obviously, please do not start eating nuts. But if you're feeling overwhelmed by giving up so many foods by choice (not by allergy), consider briefly testing the waters of an only Sugar- and Flour-free life and see how you feel. If you're this far in the book, keeping Sugar and Flour in your life is likely making your relationship with food harder, not easier. But if you want to stick to your preferences, do it with no worries—we have plenty of vegans, vegetarians, dairy-free, and pescatarian clients who are happy and successful on their terms. The choice is yours.

What about my health?

If you've read traditional diet books, you know that when trying to get as "healthy" as possible, you *must* focus on hard-core meal prep, exclusively organic food, taking supplements, eating foods at exact times, and So. Much. More. I've read more of these books than I would ever care to admit. Well, that's not exactly true. I've read the first two chapters before throwing the books against the wall in utter, overwhelming frustration.

All those rules and regulations can really make our brains shut down before we've even hit chapter three, am I right? Or worse, it results in our head in the freezer gorging on ice cream. Recommendations are only useful if we are willing to integrate them into our lives. And I don't know about you, but my life can get really *lifey* sometimes—so lifey that food prep is an impossible dream and I have to stop at a fast-food place for lunch, or that I'm eating my dinner at nine p.m. standing over my kitchen sink.

Of course, we want to be as healthy as possible. The problem we often encounter is an insistence on perfection. My stance is a little different. I want to encourage you to focus on what is realistic for your life, what minimizes harm to you, and above all, what keeps you liberated. Oddly, I've found this stance helps people to come closer to their health goals than they originally thought possible. I'm not challenging the scientific advancements in nutrition or health care; I'm challenging their unrealistic expectations of what we are sometimes capable of.

People mistakenly believe that they must purchase high-end fruit and vegetables and meal-prep every week to do the RRP successfully. That is beyond untrue. The only way this program will not work for you is if you are unwilling to break up with Sugar and Flour. The rest is negotiable—you can live a happy and healthy life eating meals out, eating lower-cost food (including fast and frozen food), not purchasing organic produce, not taking supplements, and eating dinner at eleven p.m. Are these behaviors completely ideal for our health? Probably not. Are they better than the behaviors we displayed when we were in the grip of our abusive relationship? You bet. Will these choices bring us immediate health benefits and closer to our ultimate goals, and cracking the door open to more optimal behaviors? *A thousand percent yes.*

Here's the point: *Something* is always better than nothing. And something good usually leads to more good things. Start where you are and the rest will come. Your RRP will help you navigate all of life's messy circumstances, whether they are financial restrictions, time restrictions, or willingness restrictions. And when we've solved for your restrictions, we create a more willing you—you'll be more willing to use the Instant Pot, or find room in the budget for fresh veggies, or carve out time to sit down for dinner.

WHEN AM I EATING?

In the spirit of Vow 5, "I vow to eat every 3 to 4.5 hours," I've created a plan that has you eating three meals and a snack. In my experience, I've found that eating four times a day gives your metabolism enough of a boost to help your weight release, while not taking your life hostage by requiring you to eat too often. And I really don't care how you eat your four meals: Breakfast, lunch, snack, dinner? Cool. Dinner, snack, breakfast, lunch? Fine by me. The RRP needs to fit into your life for it to be sustainable, so the combination is best dictated by you and your life.

Have you found that you're living life a little like a squirrel— snacking, grabbing, and hoarding food all day? Worried that you're not going to be full enough and that you may need a little something to hold you over? A good rule of thumb: No one ever starved to death between breakfast and lunch, snack and dinner, or dinner and breakfast. But it really may feel that way when you've given in to your hunger cues at the first sign of a tummy rumble. That's a huge part of the problem here, a part of the power that Sugar—and food in general—has over you. We need to take your power back so that food isn't stealing from your day—forcing you to leave your desk at work for a little bite of something, causing you to munch on food when you're bored (even if it's celery or carrots) or have a quick snack before you go to dinner. This messes with your already compromised hunger and fullness cues, and gives food way more power than it deserves.

If we're being honest, those tyrant-like inaccurate hunger cues that roar regardless of where you are or what you're doing are a whole lot like your relationship with Sugar, aren't they? You know what I mean: the demands to *eat now* that you instantly give in to with little and big handfuls, bits and bites that are ruling you without your consent. Not only will regulating and securing specific mealtimes help with weight release, it will also free up space in your brain and in your day to focus on creating the life you've been dreaming of.

Getting into the four-times-a-day eating schedule may be challenging at first—and rightfully so! You've been giving in to the urges, demands, and commands of Sugar and food for years and years. Putting up some boundaries will definitely come with a fight—but I promise, you are up for that fight. Punctuating your four-times-a-day eating allows for you to have a big beautiful life in between meals.

And speaking of the roar of your hunger cues, a little note on eating during the late and very early hours. For many of us, nighttime is what I like to call the "witching hour." A time when it gets very quiet outside, but often very loud inside your head. A time when you may be accustomed to drowning out the noise with Sugar, or food in general. You're in good company; I'm a recovering night eater and have helped almost every person I've treated say good-bye to the scary little gremlins that emerge at night and encourage you to chow down. If you're looking at the four-times-a-day plan and thinking, *Um, what about my nighttime ritual of eating to numb?* then we need to have a side chat here. The next chapters are all about taking food off the table as your method of coping with life, and your night-eating habit leans heavily on that crutch; it's like putting gasoline on a flame. Like Sugar, it only numbs you temporarily, and the next morning usually greets you with shame and depression, not to mention a rough time eating breakfast.

So in the many good-byes you're saying in the name of this new relationship, I encourage you to also bid farewell to night eating—it, like, Sugar, Flour, volume, and dieting, is holding you hostage. My first suggestion is to create a general time when you formally end your eating for the day. That may feel really hard in the beginning—like you need to go upstairs, lock your bedroom door, tape your mouth shut, and put cooking mitts on your hands to get through the night. And some version of that may be what you need! In my experience, it takes three solid nights without eating to regain your power—and then some maintenance along the way when the gremlins come knocking. It also may help to get some support—there are many nights I find myself texting my breaking-up-with-sugar besties, Erinn and Ali to tell them, "The kitchen is closed." Or sometimes, "The kitchen is closed with a magic lock that doesn't open until breakfast tomorrow." Or sometimes, "Kitchen closed. I'm tired not hungry."

In the spirit of "kitchen closed," I strongly advise against eating your snack after dinner or adding a snack after dinner—whatever the case may be. This after-dinner snack, as I've seen for myself and many others, can quickly become the foot in the door for a night of eating and a morning of shame. It can be a dangerous, slippery slope and the slide can happen faster than you'd believe, leading you back to food behaviors that don't work for you. Remember, the ultimate goal is to set you free. That's what you deserve. Eating at night, even if it's a snack, supports the idea that you *need* food after dinner. That's simply not true, and it's not a message we want to get behind.

HOW MUCH AM I EATING?

Vow 4 says, "I vow to be mindful of my volume." Part of truly breaking free from your destructive relationship with Sugar is releasing the weight that you've gained by overeating. Overeating *any* food—not just Sugar and Flour—certainly won't bring you the big beautiful life I've promised. The way we do that is to put some limitations on how much we eat, as absolutely heartbreaking as that may be.

There are so many conventional diet programs that talk about "free" or "unlimited" foods. While there is a case for this—yes, it is better to eat a pound of apples than a pound of doughnuts—having unlimited quantities of food doesn't help your eyes and your stomach relearn what a healthy portion of food is. Plain and simple, *the food still has the control.* And when we are creating the relationship of your dreams, we want the whole foundation to be healed, including your perception of quantity.

That's why (gasp!) I ask you to get as exact as you can about the amount of food that you're eating whenever you're able. And again, that means pulling out the measuring cups and food scale—not forever, just for right now.

You may hate me today, but you'll thank me later. Like your issue with eating four times a day, the quantity of the food and the fear that there isn't enough is absolutely hijacking your very best life. The rumble, roar, and obsession with *more* is getting in the way of all that you want and deserve. I know that with skill and faith, you can put quantity into its rightful place and be happily humming down the road to your big beautiful life.

Calorie *conscious,* not calorie *counting*

Just like not all carbs are created equal, neither are all calories. You need to upgrade your operating system if you're still living by the old-school nutrition idea of "calories in, calories out." Boy do I wish it was that simple. But the cutting-edge research shows that different food impacts our body in different ways. And different foods affect our metabolism and digestion differently, not to mention our hormones, the controller of all things hunger and fullness. Foods like your great love, Sugar, increase your appetite and cue your body to store weight, while others, like protein, increase feelings of fullness and promote weight loss. So, all calories are absolutely not created equal. Not to mention, calorie counting is one of the big culprits in your diet drama and trauma—especially your "game on" behavior when you go over your caloric allowance for the day. All that adding and subtracting steals from the big beautiful life ahead of you. You deserve *full freedom*, not another calculating and overcontrolling relationship.

And yet, there's value in knowing the "cost of a dollar" when it comes to your food, especially the costly calorically dense kind. Science says that eating fewer calories is a must in the weight-release game, so I want you to think about becoming calorie *conscious*. That means paying some attention to the caloric cost of the food that you're putting in your body. I want you to be mindful, especially with the fat and protein; be sure that you're eating them with integrity. Your RRP proteins vary widely in calorie amount—from thirty to one hundred calories per serving. And it will be no surprise to you which ones are the costly ones: cheese, nuts, eggs, and red meat—very delicious, and also very easy to overeat. The more calorically costly proteins are completely compatible with your new life, but if you're finding yourself frustrated with your weight release, they're also a likely culprit.

SUMMING IT UP

Mastering food is where the rubber really meets the road, where you will be in a position to see results in this new relationship—physically *and* emotionally. I want you to fill your life with foods that you enjoy, that you love—and that *love you back*. Back in the day, my friends would have gotten a restraining order to protect me against vanilla sheet cake if they could have. Once we've repaired and rebuilt your food foundation, we can also begin healing your life. This is where the fun begins— where we fill the space formerly reserved for cupcakes and Chinese food with new experiences, joy, fun, hobbies. And most of all, when your foundation is solid, you can get busy constructing the very best relationship with the person who matters most: *yourself.*

HOW DO I START?

Okay Molly, I'm ready. I'm ready to break up with Sugar and begin the RRP, right now. What do I do?

OMG. Yaaaaaaaaaayyyyyy! Woot! Yahoo! (Can you tell how excited I am???)

Only halfway through the book and you're ready to change your life! That's some serious courageous warrior status, my friend. Go you.

It can be pretty overwhelming and confusing starting this new relationship dance—getting the rhythm, moves, and tempo, putting one foot in front of the other in a brand-new way. I've got your back—I'm going to walk you through pre-day-one and days one, two, and three like the renegade Sherpa you've hired me to be.

Why three days? Well, mostly because a week of planning seems like a really big ask, and I know that three days of doing the dance will get you feeling hopeful enough that you'll be willing to commit to three more. I want you to start small and then build big! But if you're willing, stretch to a week of planning—and if you're type A and that feels better to you—then go on with your bad self and say seven instead of three. Let's get the party started!

Vow It: First, before you do anything, you need to head back to page 74 and review the seven vows I've laid out for you and agree to your innermost self that you can take them—even if you have to agree that you'll take them imperfectly. And, to be clear, of course I prefer you to take them 100 percent with no exception, and believe wholeheartedly that you can. Be brave.

I also need you to flip back to chapter two and review the Sacred Vow of staying the course—no cutting and running. That vow, more than the others, will come in handy in a clutch. We are really doing the thing right now, and that's going to trigger every part of you to want to cut and run, say you can't, say it's too hard, believe it's impossible. I need you to table all that noise and remember that action is the best form of persuading your thoughts to come along for the ride. It's action time.

For a minute here, we're going to need to be pretty food-focused. Remember Vow 6, "I vow to be a planner"? It's going to be key. We're going to get the basic food groundwork down so that your breakup has a soft landing.

Plan It: What do you want to eat for the next three days? Obviously, I use the term *want* loosely—you can't be having bagels and ice cream and get your breakup over and done with and your new life started. But take a look at the RRP in all its glory and figure out what you want to eat for breakfast, lunch, dinner, and snack for the first three days so we can plan accordingly. Now, if you're anything like me, the sight of sixty-six recipes may make your head spin—it's just too much. No worries. I've made you an "RRP Easy Access Cheat Sheet," which breaks down a few simple ways you can do the plan for the first few days. And listen, if you're feeling overwhelmed and nervous and just want to eat the same thing for the first week, do it—it doesn't need to be gorgeously Food Network–worthy in the beginning; it just needs to be good enough to get you through. I promise as the days pass and your head and heart heal, you'll want to venture out and add new things to the plan.

But Molly, I hate to cook and I hate to prep. And I really don't want to right now. Join the club. I never want to, so you're in good company. The truth is, if you don't want to lift a finger these first few days, you don't have to. On an "I just can't" day, I will have Starbucks Bacon and Gruyère Sous Vide Egg Bites, or pack an almond butter sandwich on Ezekiel bread (a little prep but not really); have some sort of make-your-own salad at lunch, with chicken, feta cheese, veggies, and Sugar-free dressing on the side (usually pesto vinaigrette, if you're curious); enjoy my beloved Primal Kitchen bar for snack; and order in a grilled chicken parm (weighing and eating six ounces of it) with a side salad for dinner. Of course, this lifestyle can get pricey, but so does bingeing—so maybe it's worth a little investment up front for your lifetime of peace around food.

Map It: After you've decided what you're going to eat, you need to map it. Set some time aside to write down all the food ingredients you'll need and where you'll pick them up. Then take a look at any other tools you may need—Tupperware, a nice set of knives, a spiralizer, and of course, a food scale and measuring cups.

Dump It: Then it's time to get real. And I'm going to ask you to get real in two ways. First, tell someone that you're breaking up with Sugar. Just one person. You'll learn in chapter nine how important connection is to your long-term success, and I need someone you trust and love to be there in case you need them. Effectively, this is your "in case of emergency" person. Then, I need you to make your home safe. I totally understand you have kids or roommates, or a significant other who don't have the same dysfunctional relationship with Sugar that you do—so may not be able to completely cleanse your home of all the contraband. But maybe you can! And it's my absolute wish for you. So if you can and your living-mates are on board, please do it! It will make your life sooooo much easier in the short run and the long run. No matter your situation, what you *can* do is throw away the things that really speak to you—the things that you will, despite every part of you knowing it will harm you, get you out of bed in the middle of the night for "just one." For me that would be any form of granola, any scones or shortbread cookies, and any baguette. I also have foods that I couldn't care less about—like dark chocolate, Cheez-It, and key lime pie, which I encourage my family to keep around!

Read It: Finish this book. And by that I mean read it to the very last page. I realize that you may think you're done, given you have your food plan. But that's the old way of thinking, my friend. And it's that thinking that's gotten you into your nasty relationship with dieting. This is about much more than the food. If you stop here, you're putting yourself on a diet, and that will inevitably end—and I would venture to say it will not end well. If you finish the book, I'll teach you how to create a relationship, and that will change your life. Onward.

Quick note to you, Love: Beginning this process can be daunting and also really, really tiring. You may experience detox, sadness, exhaustion, anger (all things we talk about in chapter eleven)—and that's totally normal. So to the extent that you're able, give yourself a break—try to limit the amount of parties, outings, and extracurricular things you do this week. And if you're not able to do that, then be very, *very* gentle with yourself. And know I'm here rooting for you like my life depends on it.

The Cheat Sheet below and Relationship Rebuild Food Plan in the appendix give you the broad strokes of how to structure your meals every day. The Cheat Sheet is a quick and easy reference guide, pulled from the larger RRP, while the RRP is a deeper dive into all the options for your meals and snacks. Again, the long-form version of your amazing Relationship Rebuild Food Plan and more easy meal concepts and recipes, can be found Appendix B.

RRP EASY ACCESS CHEAT SHEET

Reminder: These food choices are examples, not what you're "supposed" to eat. Don't like them? Head to the recipe section of the Relationship Rebuild Food Plan and see what works for you!

Breakfast Concepts

(A) *2 servings Protein + 1 serving Carbohydrate + 1 serving Fruit or Fat*

2 eggs (cooked any way you want!) + 1 piece toasted Ezekiel bread + ¾ cup berries or ⅓ medium avocado

---

(B) *2 servings Protein + 2 servings Carbohydrate*

2 tablespoons almond butter + 2 pieces toasted Ezekiel bread

(C) *3 servings Protein + 1 serving Carbohydrate or Fruit*

3 eggs (cooked any way you want!) + 1 Ezekiel wrap or 1 whole (6-ounce) apple

---

Lunch Concepts

(A) *3–5 servings Protein + 1 serving Carbohydrate + 1 serving Fat + Veggies**

6 ounces tuna packed in water + 1 Ezekiel wrap + 1 tablespoon mayo + lettuce and tomato

---

(B) *3 servings Protein + 1–2 servings Carbohydrate + 1 serving Fat + Veggies**

6 ounces white-meat chicken + ½–⅔ cup rice and beans + ⅓ medium avocado + chopped tomato

---

(C) *3–5 servings Protein + 2 servings Fat + Veggies**

5 ounces salmon + 2 tablespoons Caesar dressing (regular fat) + 2 cups romaine lettuce

---

Snack Concepts

(A) *2 servings Protein + 1 serving Fruit/ Veggies**

1 cup unsweetened 2 percent yogurt + 1 chopped apple + cinnamon

2 low-fat cheese sticks + 3 ounces banana (½ medium banana)

(B) *2 servings Fat + Veggies**

6 tablespoons guacamole + 1 cup carrot sticks

(C) *2 servings Protein + 1 serving Carbohydrate*
2 tablespoons natural almond butter + 1 piece toasted Ezekiel bread

---

Dinner Concepts

(A) *3–5 servings Protein + 1 serving Carbohydrate + 1 serving
  Fat + Veggies**
5 ounces roasted dark-meat chicken + 1 small sweet potato
  (4 ounces) + 1 tablespoon butter + steamed bag of veggies

(B) *3 servings Protein + 1–2 servings Carbohydrate + 1 serving
  Fat + Veggies**
Fish Tacos: 6 ounces tilapia + ½ cup cooked brown rice + 1
  tablespoon ranch dressing + shredded lettuce, tomato, and onion

---

(C) *3–5 servings Protein + 2 servings Fat + Veggies**
*3–5 ounces ground beef + 1 tablespoon olive oil +
  3 tablespoons sour cream + zoodles mixed with tomato
  sauce and beef*

I Broke Up with Sugar

Camille

I have been on and off diets since probably the age of thirteen, and I
have always had a love-hate relationship with food. I would experience
a horrible cycle of bingeing, shame, bingeing again, and dealing with
more shame! For so long, I never realized I was in an abusive
relationship with Flour and Sugar that was fueling the need for
volume. That is, until I broke it off and kicked Flour and Sugar to the
curb. In the past, the more I ate, the more I needed to consume to get
that "high." My binges were so focused and determined!

Once I got rid of Sugar and Flour, my body started to get the cues back to let me know when I was full and when I was truly hungry. I was able to take a step back and see what I was doing—my body was recalibrating. My mind still wanted Sugar and Flour, but without all those chemicals swirling in my system, I could take a step back and make better decisions. My body started to feel better, the cobwebs from my brain started to clear, and I started to see that this image I had of how I wanted my life to be was in fact possible!

It can be hard to give up your source of comfort, but it is not impossible and the rewards are mind-blowing. There has been such a spiritual component to this journey. The concept of consciously living my life with integrity is something that has always been missing. It has really made me look at my life and how I want it to look. What started out as a very desperate attempt to lose weight has turned into this life-changing new relationship with food.

I Broke Up with Sugar

Tracy

Before breaking up with Sugar, my life was a roller coaster. I have been on diets for as long as I can remember. I remember bringing strange diet food to school as a kid; one diet was hard-boiled eggs, beets, and ice cream—no joke. I used juice cleanses like a Band-Aid, or even as a punishment, after a binge episode. There were diets in which I only ate steamed vegetables and drank green juices. I was *terrified* of fats, I avoided carbs, ate portions no bigger than the size of my fist, and worked out almost every day. I called the gym the "calorie bank" and kept track of how many calories I ate and how many I burned at the gym. My weight was always fluctuating by about fifty pounds, up or down. The whole thing was totally unsustainable.

Sometimes I could lose the weight, but it always crept back on during dark times. I relied on food for coping with stress, sadness, anxiety, and exhaustion and for seeking comfort, companionship, avoidance, and so much more. Along with this was the belief system that was ingrained in my head for my whole life: *I am fat. I am ugly. I am unlovable*. I used up every birthday wish year after year on *I wish to lose weight*. I always believed that if I lost weight, I'd be happy, as if the weight was my one and only barrier to happiness.

Before I started this program, I was eating vegan "health" foods, working out, and still gaining weight. I was frustrated and didn't understand what was wrong, so I went to nutritionist after nutritionist, looking for answers. Then one day four years ago, I met Molly. She looked me dead in the eye and simply said, "It's the Sugar." I argued with her that it was impossible because I only ate vegan health food. She taught me the more than fifty different names for hidden sugars and sent me back out there to read labels in a more educated way. That's how I learned that there was Sugar in *everything* I was eating—I had no idea. And that's when I finally saw the light in terms of my lifelong struggle with food. What I needed to do was avoid Sugar and Flour.

Ultimately, I learned the most about how Sugar affects the body, mind, and spirit by giving it up myself and witnessing what happened. What's more, doing the plan gave a ceiling to the endless noise in my brain about when and what to eat. People like me have constant brain chatter: *Should I eat that? Am I hungry? Why did I eat that? I'm still hungry. I shouldn't eat that.* The snacking, grazing, bingeing, shaming . . . now suddenly it was all simplified: This is what you eat, this is when you eat, and that's that. Early on when I was doing the program, I remember wondering what I would do with all the newly available brain space. I needed that structure. And I believe that without the Sugar and Flour in my body, which are highly addictive, I am able to follow my food plan. And ironically, my food tastes a lot better since giving up Sugar. I was avoiding fats and seasonings for years because I was afraid of them being "fattening." Now I know what foods I can eat safely that add flavor and excitement to my food. And honestly, my palate has changed without Sugar. I am proof that a vegan can successfully be Sugar- and Flour-free.

Yes, I lost weight once the Sugar and Flour were out of my body. But perhaps the biggest change was in my mind and spirit. About sixty days after I gave up Sugar, I thought I was going crazy. I felt so much more energy and a more positive outlook on life, and I walked through the world with more ease. I actually had a friend ask me what type of antianxiety medication I was on because she noticed my anxiety was alleviated. I remember thinking, *Wow, after thirty-eight years of life on this planet, I am only now learning how to love myself for the first time.*

Molly's program brought me salvation and peace from the torture of dieting and a lifelong struggle with food and weight. Four years later, I am still following my food plan, but I am also living a big beautiful life with no restrictions. Once you learn how to navigate it, you can do it almost without thinking. But for my food to be in order, I have to keep up the self-care and continue my journey working on what's behind the food. I am committed to remaining Sugar-free because there's no piece of cake that tastes good enough for me to go back to the way I was living before I gave up Sugar.

I Broke Up with Sugar

Robin

I started the program with Molly because after years of not having to worry about my weight, I found myself at a weight I had never seen before. I was eating more Sugar and Flour than before and was not able to stop. The program was simple and made sense: Take out the things I can't control portions of—the foods that I continually overate; I had to break up with Sugar and Flour. My plan allows almost *everything* else with lots of wiggle room. I love everything I eat and am always (healthfully) excited for my meals!

What was most unexpected for me was the result. It was far more than just releasing weight—I discovered a better, energized, focused me. Molly helped me to break up with the foods I loved that didn't love me back. I'm now able to eat with complete freedom. I said good-bye to the cravings and mood swings and welcomed a balanced and awakened new version of myself. My sixties really are my new forties (I really wouldn't want the twenties or thirties; they come with too much drama).

Chapter 8

Real Talk: What to Do When Sugar Comes Crawling Back (And You Know It Will)

Breaking up is hard to do. You already know this. But you might not have known just how hard until this breakup with Sugar. And while this uncoupling is *wonderful and freeing*—opening your eyes to a life you didn't even know was possible—it's also left you pretty lost and empty. So, what are you going to do without your lover and best friend?

I can guarantee that Sugar is going to make every attempt to weasel back in and fill this void. If you think this is going to be one of those clean breaks, where you never see Sugar again, you're seriously underestimating its power and persistence. And why *wouldn't* it think it still had a shot? For . . . well, *forever*, you've been eating to meet all your needs—physical, emotional, and everything in between. Without question, you're going to have cravings and urges that will make you want to run—scratch that, *sprint* straight back to Sugar's toxic embrace when the going gets tough.

We need to address the obvious issue that's been completely overlooked in your previous attempts to deal with this relationship, before you knew the real deal. That issue, my friends, is *life*. It's going to be hard, difficult feelings are going to surface, and life is going to get *lifey*—we both know that. As of now, your default reaction is to turn to your relationship with Sugar for comfort.

Because you've consistently turned to Sugar when life gets depressing and tough, and also when it gets joyful and happy—so really, all the time—you've gotten trapped in a pretty nasty cycle. Sugar's your go-to for all situations, good and bad. And as a result, it's stolen all your power and made you believe you're fragile and can't deal without it. You are *far* from fragile. You are strong, you are capable, you are a warrior! Your reliance on Sugar and Flour has made you forget your true nature. It has clouded your mind, dulled your senses, and blurred your vision.

This is the part of your journey where the change really happens. It's sort of like learning to write with your left hand if you're a righty—not easy but totally possible, and eventually natural. Your tendency to rely on Sugar to cope with life is the biggest problem on your relationship plate right now. It's the barrier between you and what you want. And I'm not understating it. You actually can't start living this big beautiful life that you deserve while you're still in your dysfunctional relationship with Sugar.

But *no worries*. I've got your back! With a little information and *a lot* of direction, we'll have you ignoring the flowers, love notes, and (empty) promises Sugar's famous for when trying to regain entry into your life. Before you know it, you'll be making strides toward a new, empowered, and sustainable way of living your life.

CRAVINGS ARE NOT COMMANDS

Sugar cravings can be beyond overwhelming. It's like the devil is possessing you and screaming, "YOU NEED TO EAT RIGHT NOW!" It feels like all control has vanished and you *have* to eat. And while you may not believe it right now, research shows this is the furthest thing from the truth. Cravings can make you feel crazy—like they completely dominate you. Good news, though: Cravings give you many opportunities to seize the steering wheel. It's time to take back your power!

When cravings come and you consider *not* turning to Sugar, it can cause you to become reactive and demand that the cravings go away—*now*! This is the most ineffective thing you can do; trying to make a craving go away is like trying to control the ocean. It's not possible.

And when you're not a skilled ocean swimmer, waves smack against your face and the undertow drags you down—just like cravings do.

When you become more experienced with the ocean's surges, you learn how to anticipate the waves, ride them, and make them work for you. And every single time, they crash and mellow out. Same with your cravings—we just need to teach you how to tolerate them, how to surf your urges. Because research tells us that even though they totally feel like they are going to last forever, cravings are episodic, not constant, and they rarely last more than thirty minutes. And here we are giving in to them, letting them exhaust us and make us feel hopeless, when all we really need to do is learn how to give them time to pass.

Effectively, your cravings for Sugar are exactly like Sugar—they get stronger and stronger every time you feed them, like pouring gasoline on a flame. Cravings are like little kids—they scream and hold their breath in the middle of the floor demanding a cupcake: "I want it! I want it! I want it! Noooooowwwwwww!" And when you always give in, you're reinforcing and rewarding your craving's temper tantrums.

But lucky for us, the opposite is also completely true: If you don't give in to your cravings, they become less and less frequent. Cue the same kid melting down over a cupcake. If you don't give in, eventually, the kid starts to learn that tantrums aren't an effective way to get treats, and the tantrums become weaker and less frequent (that's a lot of energy to spend for no cupcake!).

So while we can't control the thoughts that pop into our heads, we *can* control our actions. Just because we feel the urge to eat everything right this second doesn't mean we need to do it. And the less we act on those impulses, the more our brains learn that cravings don't manifest cupcakes . . . or unnecessary dopamine spikes.

I know you're sitting there saying, "No way, Molly. Not possible. You cannot begin to understand how intense my cravings are." Don't knock it till you've tried it—I was once the queen of doubt about this . . . *until I did it.*

My old therapist once urged me to try riding out a craving, explaining to me that people don't always "go home and eat their entire refrigerator." This was fascinating news! In fact, she said, people go home, put on their pajamas, wash their faces, and watch television. And so I went home that night, scared of all the demons that would start chatting with me. Boy was it was weird to go home and resist the cabinet—without tearing through a bag of chips followed by ice cream and so much more. But like a soldier, I got home, went to my bedroom, put on my pj's, washed my face, put on an episode of *ER*, and eventually went to sleep, without Sugar to knock me out. It was well over a decade ago, and I can still remember it: the very first time I challenged food and won.

Not every attempt was this seamless—sometimes things got ugly, complete with literal sweat and tears. Eventually, though, by not giving in and not surrendering to Sugar, I found it became pretty common to successfully surf my cravings.

Yeah, Molly, good for you. You're amazing and can beat your urges. Not me. Cravings are not commands. That sentence may not feel true, but you can make it real. Research shows that when we eat the foods we crave less frequently (Ummmmm, hello Sugar and Flour!), our cravings for that food decrease. So you see, you have all the power to ride out these cravings and take back your control.

FEELINGS PHOBIC

Ah, the evil f-word: feelings. You've been turning to Sugar at the slightest hint of a feeling. And just like giving in to cravings, numbing your feelings keeps you locked in this relationship. We numb what we don't want to feel. Stressful day at work? Pour yourself a few glasses of wine when you get home and forget about it, until your hangover the next morning. Feeling isolated from your partner? Hop online for some "retail therapy," feeling the thrill of new stuff, but also racking up your credit card debt. Same with Sugar—pick up a few cupcakes and a pint of ice cream after being denied a promotion; it's your escape route from all the feelings.

Feelings are actually a very important part of being human, FYI. They are necessary to our survival! They let us know when things are warm, good, and safe, and they deter and protect us from the things that are not. Feelings are incredibly useful. But by using food to deal with life, you've short-circuited the system and your feelings are no longer allowed to do their job. And it may be contributing to why your life isn't feeling as warm, good, or safe as you wish it did.

Worst of all, when Sugar is numbing your painful feelings, it's erasing your ability to experience pleasure. Your brain cannot engage in either direction—positive or negative—when it's numbed out, which means you're missing out on the happiness, joy, love, satisfaction, and fun that life has to offer. And that's no good. Let me promise you, with all the love in my heart, if you think your life has no promise of joy, you are dead wrong. I have seen so many clients who didn't believe they could be happy, who didn't understand how anyone walked down the street with any level of contentment. And when they found their new relationship with food and with themselves, that tune changed quickly.

Learning to truly feel your emotions is super important. While feelings may seem to last forever, it's not actually as long as you might think. Learning how to manage them isn't necessarily the most fun thing you can do on a Saturday afternoon, but you also get a new idea of your own strength when you're less afraid of negative feelings arising. Not to mention, there are proven and healthy strategies to decrease the duration and intensity of uncomfortable feelings, like practicing mediation, distracting, and self-soothing (more on these fantastic tools in the next chapter). Know for now that feelings—good and bad—always, always, always pass if you let them. And they certainly won't kill you in the process, I promise. Your job is to manage them without running to the kitchen.

Once you stop using food to numb yourself, you may notice a brief but rudely unpleasant surge of emotions. It's almost like turning on a stopped-up rusty faucet—dark brown, foul-smelling water gushes out in uneven spurts, but eventually the water will run clear. Same thing when you stop numbing your feelings with Sugar and Flour: Your distressing feelings will come—perhaps also dark brown and putrid—in the first weeks post-breakup. But I can attest that it will not be like this forever. Far from it! In fact, after this rough patch you'll start having more genuine positive feelings and experiences than you ever had while you were in an abusive relationship with Sugar and Flour.

PUTTING ON MY THERAPIST HAT

Yes, feelings pass. Yes, you can and *need to* gain skills to learn how to manage your feelings and not let them manage you. But sometimes, especially if you've suffered in the worst and darkest parts of this abusive relationship, breaking up can reveal things that you may not be equipped to deal with. While your toolbox can help to manage these issues and insights, you may want to look into getting some additional support to help you heal. Outside support can look like individual or group therapy, getting more involved in your spiritual life, or finding a self-help group that can work on the issues that come up outside of your relationship with Sugar and Flour.

THE POWER OF COPING SKILLS: SUGAR IS NOT A SKILL

I'm probably not the first person who's ever suggested that you get a toolbox and start using healthy coping skills when cravings crop up or when you're having uncomfortable feelings. I may be the first person who makes a case for this in a way that gets you to do it, though. Fingers crossed.

What, exactly, are coping skills? Plain and simple, they are the behaviors and actions you can develop that help you to manage emotions and that get you through difficult and challenging times. They allow you to stay true to all the things you want in your big beautiful life. Coping skills are techniques such as distracting yourself with a crossword, chatting with a friend, taking an ice cold or hot shower, singing at the top of your lungs, smelling flowers in the park, or taking deep breaths. More on these in the next chapter.

I'm not saying this is easy—especially with the attachment you have to Sugar—but having these new tools is essential in building the solid foundation you need to succeed in the new life you're building. When I say essential, I mean *essential*.

I need you to understand and start to accept this hard truth: *Sugar is not a skill.* As of now, your go-to coping skill for tolerating uncomfortable feelings and managing hard times is Sugar. You've become accustomed to numbing your feelings, particularly the awful ones, through the use of food. This would be a solution made in heaven, if not for one critical pitfall: It's absolutely unsustainable. And it's making and keeping you miserable.

If nothing changes, nothing changes

Clearly you need to learn a better way to manage hard feelings and cravings. Because when you lean on Sugar to do it, not only do you cue the feelings of failure and demoralization, you also reinforce your cravings, making them more frequent and intense.

You're a veteran of diet wars if you've been on . . . let's say five diets. I'm sure there are many of you laughing, thinking, *Five! Try five thousand!* And if this is you, then the topic of skills is not an unfamiliar one. It's one of the most important topics in this book—and the one to which we are usually the most resistant.

Yes, I see you rolling your eyes. I know it sounds like these skills are no match for the hole that Sugar has left in your life. But we're at a serious turning point here. When the cravings come, you can choose to turn back to Sugar and . . . well, you know the rest, *or* you can try this new idea I'm presenting you. The choice is yours. (Please try it!) And truth be told, you're not the first one to protest using these skills. You're probably thinking, *There's no way these skills will help me feel better. It will take too long. I'll get too impatient. I hate watercolors. And there's absolutely no way this will work as well as Sugar, or be enough to get me through tough times. I'll still turn to the Sugar afterward, so what's the point?*

Boy, do I get it. I can't tell you the number of conventional diet programs, weight-loss groups, nutritionists, and therapists that have tried to get this point across to me! It was in one ear and right out the other. Sure, I understood the concept, but the food was Just. So. Comforting. And the idea of painting with watercolors or doing self-massage felt beyond useless when I could count on my greatest love, Sugar, to get me through.

My mind was changed when I started training with one of my beloved teachers, Dr. Marsha Linehan. I am not understating it when I say she is an actual genius. Dr. Linehan developed dialectical behavioral therapy (DBT), which is one of the most researched and evidence-based behavioral treatment models to date. DBT has helped people to decrease their suicide attempts by 70 percent, among a whole host of other incredible outcomes. It's also been shown to be incredibly effective for both addiction and eating disorders. Dr. Linehan subscribes so wholeheartedly to the concept of skills that she devotes almost a quarter of her treatment model to what she calls *distress tolerance*—learning how to let painful feelings and experiences pass without making them worse. It was this quote that she shared in her teachings that really turned me:

> *Distress tolerance, at least over the short run, is part and parcel of any attempt to change oneself; otherwise, impulsive actions will interfere with efforts to establish desired changes.*

Marsha Linehan does not mince words. This is a very scholarly way of saying that while food is still on the table as an option to soothe you in good times and in bad, it is going to be literally impossible for you to make the changes we've been talking about. As long as Sugar—or food in general—is still in your how-to-deal-with-life toolbox, these other skills will *never work*. And I'm talking about *all* food. If you offer me a choice of eating carrots or listening to music, I'm always going to go with crunching on carrots. And carrots lead to apples lead to protein bars lead to candy bars, so food—*all* food—needs to be removed from your toolbox. They say in the recovery communities, "If nothing changes, nothing changes." And we are here to change *every* part of your relationship with food and with yourself.

Great Expectations

Michael, a client of mine, really hated this idea. Over and over for an entire session, he screamed at me, "But Molly, nothing will ever work like the food! Nothing will ever feel as good!" Finally, I looked at him and said, "Yes, Mike. Nothing will ever feel as good as the food. But nothing will ever feel as bad." #truthbomb

When times get rough, some people think about taking a relaxing bubble bath—but not you, because bubble baths don't feel like Sugar! That's true. And it's also true that we have an expectation problem on our hands. Remember in chapter three when I taught you about how Sugar cues your dopamine, which launches you into a never-ending cycle of trying to feel good? In the maintenance and pursuit of this effect—that is, feeling good or not feeling at all, and in the face of negative feelings—you're creating an expectation of how you're supposed to tolerate pain, of how a skill should work. Your concept of success is feeling numbed out and totally forgetting everything . . . including the demoralization the next day.

So what's to be expected of this new toolbox you are about to create? **The only expectation you can have of a skill is that it helps you to tolerate the moment without making it worse.** Whoa. We're going to need to put a capital *R* on Realistic here, because your expectations are definitely out of whack. That means if you're feeling bereft and sad and you watch a movie to take your mind off things (a.k.a. tolerate the moment), you may still feel the sadness after the movie, *but you haven't made the moment worse by turning to Sugar.* You haven't perpetuated the negative cycle of turning to Sugar and food to make things temporarily better, only to feel hopeless and hungover in the morning, adding more problems and drama to the sadness you started with. Make sense?

There are times when using a coping skill can simply help to pass the time, giving you some space to exercise your best judgment to say no to Sugar. Once in a while using a skill can improve your mood, but that's kind of an added bonus. The goal of using a skill is to get through the tough moment without turning to Sugar. You might still feel sad afterward, but you're definitely not also in a shame cycle after downing a box of cookies. What really matters is avoiding making icky situations more icky. If your skill has helped you accomplish this, then a big *V* for victory!

I Broke Up with Sugar

Karyn

Food and weight have been an issue my entire life. I was a heavy child. Food for me was not just substance to survive. It became a *relationship*, a crutch for all emotions—happy, sad, frustrated. And Sugar affected every aspect of my life. I lost weight prior to high school and kept it off for some time, but when my mother died, I gained 120 pounds that year, without even realizing it.

I played the dieting game for more than thirty years. I was on Weight Watchers, I did South Beach, I ate only nine grams of carbs a day. It was completely unsustainable. My weight was up and down. I would think I was doing well starving myself and then life would happen, and I would flip back into bingeing in the blink of an eye. Cheat days didn't work for me, either, in the same way cheat days don't work for an alcoholic. I experienced such shame and disgust in the dieting cycle I entered again and again. It was a constant battle, and all my dieting fiascoes were bringing me further and further away from a life of recovery and peace.

The last straw was after I had an accidental fall and sustained an injury at work. I had gained so much weight, and depression started to kick in. I ate and ate because I couldn't move. And as I kept gaining weight, my family was pleading with me to stop. I was spiraling out of control.

When I met Molly, I was at my rock bottom. She told me about my abusive relationship with Sugar and Flour. It was hard to accept, but I soon realized I was an addict. I told her I was ready to change, without really knowing what I was ready for. At first, the program felt like a diet because it was such a huge change. The first part was tough. I went through withdrawal and grief. I cried thinking about Thanksgiving coming up and not eating my favorite pecan pie. But soon after starting the program, I started to think of my breakup with Sugar and Flour as my new life, not a deprivation diet or a punishment. I soon realized I didn't miss Sugar at all! Letting go of Sugar has been such a relief; my shame and self-hate are gone! When a craving comes to me now, I place my hand over my heart and ask myself, "What am I really feeling?" I've learned not to sabotage myself. I am able to focus so much better and feel confident, as if I'm winning a race. I no longer have that monster on my back now that Sugar and Flour are out of my life.

My attitude about dieting has also changed. I learned that if I mess up one day, I forgive myself and move on. I practice flexibility, encourage myself, and feel strong emotionally. I deal with things now; I don't just push them down with food. My family is so happy to see the change in me, and I can finally be active with my grandchild. I practice prayer, gratitude, and meditation throughout my day. Molly's guidance has really helped me tremendously. I can walk again, and my inflammation is mostly gone. I love the food I eat, and I no longer have cravings for sweet things. I've lost eighty-five pounds so far. I still have more to go, and I'm so optimistic about my journey. I feel like I have all the tools to continue on my path of recovery now.

Chapter 9

Filling That Gaping Hole:
Skills for Mind, Body, and Spirit

I f you want to know why you're in a destructive relationship with Sugar and Flour, stop eating them and you'll figure it out pretty quickly. Beyond a shadow of doubt, leaving this relationship will be one of the best things you'll ever do for yourself—and I mean *ever*. But as the process of learning how to live without the foods you've used to cope unfolds, you're probably going to feel some serious emptiness or some serious craziness—in either case, like a gaping hole has been dug in your soul. Let's start talking about filling it.

You've been barely surviving in an abusive relationship with food for a while now, using it to quell your pain and numb out—and it's been leaving you worse off in the long run. Now you're being given a chance to replace these coping mechanisms with skills that expand and augment your life, instead of things that deplete your spirit and keep you trapped in this damaging cycle. It's a call for celebration! So let's work on shifting your perspective . . . fast!

THE DOUBTING OF THE DIET VETERAN

I remember very early in my career I was treating a woman, Betty, a longtime diet war veteran who could not stop eating at night. And it was always the same scenario: She was home, feeling lonely and overwhelmed, she heard the cookies in the cabinet whispering promises of numbness and relief, so she ate the bag, and woke up in the morning feeling worse than when she started. Over and over. Night after night.

I gently suggested to Betty that we may want to find her a nightly distraction—a way to tolerate her unpleasant feelings without making them worse. Like a bubble bath, a hand massage, really trashy TV, you know the deal. And whoa. Betty came at me like a tiger! "What! A bubble bath? Are you freaking kidding, Molly? I thought you really got me and here you are suggesting I take a stupid bubble bath just like every other person I've ever seen for my food problems!" Angrily, she grabbed her coat and started to put it on. I looked at her and softly said, "Betty. Have you ever *tried* a bubble bath? There's really good research that says it may help with this pain you're in." She stared at me in shock and said, "No. I haven't," took her coat off, and said, "Tell me more."

Betty's story is all our stories. You're not a real diet veteran if you haven't rolled your eyes or vehemently argued that a bubble bath won't help your food problem. Like I told you—I was the doubtingest of the diet veterans. I would have gleefully worn a T-shirt proclaiming "Skills Don't Work" given my feelings on the topic.

As we learned in the previous chapter, it doesn't matter if you *want* to fill up this toolbox, the fact is you *need* to if your sincere goal is to break up with Sugar and reclaim your relationship with food and with yourself. It's time to get over this uncompromising view of using skills . . . now. Because we're sitting here looking at your sad little toolbox, with Sugar and Flour as its only inhabitants, and that simply will not work.

You need new ways to deal with uncomfortable feelings and cravings. Ones that love you back. Techniques that don't lead to crazy insulin spikes, intense dopamine rushes, and exhausting blood-sugar crashes. Skills that don't leave you wallowing in self-loathing at the end of the day, but instead leave you feeling nurtured, balanced, and ready to take on life.

If you're up for it—and you *are*, you warrior—we're going to put together the fanciest, most cutting-edge toolbox around, one that helps to alleviate your pain in the moment and empowers you to stay calm, cool, and collected while you're rocking your new life.

STABLE IS THE NEW SEXY

We can agree that your relationship with food has been rocky, to say the least—with crazy highs and terrifying lows. One day you're binge-ing on pints of ice cream; the next you're groaning in self-loathing, swearing to yourself *this* will be the first day of your new life, only to find yourself locked back in the cycle by sundown. We've got to get you out of this soul-crushing predicament.

In order to do that, you're going to have to embrace a new way of thinking and living. Food can't be so sexy. It can no longer provide all this excitement and sense of risk and adventure. By removing Sugar and Flour's death grip on your life, you'll be able to reap exhilaration and joy from *your actual life*. That's the gift that keeps on giving.

Can we get honest? Stomach bloat, hangover haze, and paralyzing shame aren't exactly sexy—by *Vogue*'s standards or anyone else's. You know what is? Stability. People are endlessly striving to release weight and establish a healthy relationship with food. And here you are, ac-complishing it! And I know that the more balanced and secure your skill set and life become, the easier this will be. Last time I checked, becoming the reliable, confident, and self-assured person you're trans-forming into is *by definition* sexy.

That being said, taking out the highs and lows that come with using food as your go-to skill will require some effort. And given that your brain is conditioned to reach for food when things get tough, it proba-bly won't feel all that sexy at first. But over time and with practice using your new, shiny cutting-edge skills, you'll be strutting through life with a glimmer in your eye, walking on your path to freedom. You're bring-ing sexy back!

GET YOUR DANCE CARD READY:
DATING THE SKILLS

Now, neither one of us is crazy enough to think that you're just going to go and use a coping skill the first time things feel hard, when you've never done it before. Right? When you're feeling all the feels and it's really bad, your most familiar action is to *eat*. And, sadly, your brain can reach a tipping point where I could be standing in your kitchen asking if you wanted to try using a skill and you'd snarl and barrel right through me to get to the chocolate. That's what an abusive relationship with Sugar does—it isn't personal; I'd do the same to you.

You're never going to turn to a skill when you're on fire, unless you first learn to use them when you're chilled out. That's why getting to know these skills, trying them on for size, seeing how you feel about them—*dating* these skills (with potential for a long-term relationship, of course)—is an absolutely crucial part of creating your toolbox and your new relationship with food.

It's also an essential part of creating your new relationship with yourself. In its pillage and plunder of your spirit, Sugar has stolen some of your sense of self, muddying your likes and dislikes. Dating the skills is a 1 + 1 = 3 situation, giving you a chance to create new ways to tolerate hard times and also to learn what excites you, create new experiences, and help you to really know yourself. That's what I call a win-win-win.

It's time to date your skills. Every single week I need you to give a few new ones a chance, encourage the ones that are working for you, and let the ones that aren't working for you down easily, so that when the tough times come—and you know they will—you have your tried-and-true skills to rely on and support you.

SO MANY SKILLS, SO LITTLE TIME

Listen, I'm here to help you rewire this whole operation so that you start thinking of something other than Sugar when you find yourself in a bind. And if you don't think I'm going to give you a Fourth of July Spectacular presentation of all the skills, then you underestimate me. I'm going to parade a lot of options before you, because I want you to have the fanciest, most fly toolbox around. But I don't want you to be overwhelmed by all the suitor-skills knocking on your door, so I made you a Skills Calling Card, which you can find in the appendix of this book. Your Calling Card will help you to keep track of all the skills you've tried, whether you like them, and whether you'd like to date them again. Remember, more is more when it comes to the skills game, and there's no such thing as promiscuity, so try a lot and love a lot!

May I please introduce you to . . . your skills

Enough of all this talk about why this is so important—let's get to the business of action. Let's get you acquainted with your new potential skills—the crucial components of the beautiful life you are creating.

There are two kinds of skills you'll need to have in your toolbox:

Right-Now Skills: For when life is beating up on you and you don't want to make a bad situation worse by turning to Sugar and Flour. These will be your on-the-go, quick-and-dirty ways of managing your life instead of letting your life manage you.

Long-Lasting Skills: These skills will form a bulletproof infrastructure that will make your friends jealous! Seriously, employing these skills will not only make your mind, body, and spirit stronger, you'll also become more flexible and resilient, which will allow you to bounce back to your best self—faster and more often.

Important announcement! I need you to remember your first vow: *Keep an open mind.* Don't pull a Betty. Trying new things can shut down even the most willing of minds. If these skills are going to work for you—and they *are* going to work for you—you need to get curious about them and figure out the ways they're going to support you. In short, don't knock it 'til you've tried it—over and over and over.

Right-Now Skills

Life can really get lifey, that's for sure. And if you're going to live a big beautiful one, the lifeyness will abound. There will be times when you're going to feel intense and uncomfortable emotions, which may trigger strong urges to eat. It's part of the deal. Life can make you want to scream at the top of your lungs or into the bottom of a gallon of ice cream. Oh, I get it. And given that your knee-jerk reaction is to use Sugar, we need to introduce you to some new ASAP skills . . . ASAP. Meet your Right-Now Skills.

Dealing with distress . . . and not making things worse

Discomfort will come in all shapes and sizes. When it does, your skills are going to help you to learn to embrace the old adage "This too shall pass." Operative word: *learn*. Right now, while you're passing the time waiting for a hard moment to end, you're doing it elbow deep in a bag of candy, which is making things worse, not better.

We need to turn you into an expert at passing time when you're feeling uncomfortable—whether it's from a Sugar craving, a deep feeling of grief, work drama, an outfit not looking right, or even just bumper-to-bumper traffic when you're running late. Because none of those things last forever, and when you can tolerate unpleasant moments in a healthy way, you leave the experience with the strength of knowing your own tenacity. This is how you achieve resilience—the superpower ability to bounce back. You develop resilience by leaning on healthy skills when times get tough. And remember, urges and difficult feelings are only temporary, I promise; they always pass. Your goal is not to force them to go away, but instead to find ways to take your mind off them while they are doing their thing, which helps to make them tolerable.

Quick reminder: Every time you turn to Sugar to quell, soothe, or help you tolerate a craving or an uncomfortable feeling, you're teaching your brain that you can't tolerate it and that Sugar needs to come to your rescue. That's taking a big step backward instead of propelling yourself forward toward your new life.

How do I pass the time when I'm by myself?

Being uncomfortable when you're alone can be very dark and stormy. It's where Sugar sings its enchanting song, making you feel like it's your best and only choice. Take note, it's definitely not. Enter the most underrated skill around: distraction. Distraction has been used since we were very young. Think of sad and angry little kids who are suddenly smiling at a joke their parents tell, or giggling at a little tickle. We can re-create this childhood experience as adults by focusing our attention on somewhere other than the source of our discomfort, letting it pass with more ease. You may not be giggling in your bedroom while Sugar is demanding you go downstairs and eat, but if you can find the right methods, you actually might! Videos of babies eating lemons? Hilarious. Getting down and deep into a new mystery novel? Riveting. Neither your cup of tea? No problem. Lucky for you, distractions are plentiful. Get into a TV series, start knitting or crafting, google anything and get lost in it, listen or dance to music, take a walk outside, check in on your best friend. Literally anything that occupies your mind or body—anything except stuffing your face, that is—is fair game.

How do I distract myself when I'm with a bunch of people?

Being around people—at work, on family vacations, out to dinner—can feel more restrictive when it comes to tolerating your distress. When you're in a business meeting and you're unable to break eye contact with the doughnuts on the table, it's not like you can whip out a watercolor project, make a cup of tea, or start playing a game on your phone. Don't fret—this is a solvable problem. There are skills you probably didn't realize are available when you're not flying solo.

Your imagination is the very best tool in these situations. And you're in good company. Highly competitive athletes, boxers, runners, soccer players, and gymnasts all use this skill to navigate and overcome potential obstacles that may come their way; they visualize their ideal performance. And when they use this skill it works! Visualization leads to better performance and success. Imagine getting through the meeting without eating the doughnut, how amazing you'll feel when the trying time is over. What about imagining your very favorite place on earth—like the forest or the beach? Or conjuring up an image of your favorite person or animal? Remember, we need to create a distraction to get us through the moment—and these images can really do the trick.

My very favorite skill—especially when I'm having a craving and getting away from the food is in my best interest—is to take a time-out . . . in the bathroom. I take a little break, splash some cold water on my face, or wash my hands really vigorously with very cold or very hot water. And I almost always am able to return to the situation with a better perspective.

Skills to soothe your inner savage beast

I love a good distraction when it comes to using skills, but I *really* love a good soothe when my cravings are screaming like little beasts. And as it turns out, our senses are super receptive and a great pathway to helping us calm down. Self-massage, listening to music, enjoying some tea, taking a hot shower or luxurious bubble bath, using a weighted blanket, experimenting with essential oils, doing an at-home facial, smelling flowers, snuggling with your pet or partner, looking at beautiful art, lighting candles, squeezing a stress ball, taking a walk in the park or in nature—without food running the show, you have so much space and time to try new things to make you calm and tranquil.

A second plug for opening your mind

I have clients who have fallen head over heels for bath bombs and adult coloring books, and others who have become podcast connoisseurs and seekers of hilarious YouTube videos. I myself am a Spotify-listening, necklace-crafting, bath-taking, tea-drinking, skill-loving lunatic in the best way possible! All of us would have bet against the idea of skills being useful, and all of us would say today that these skills have been key to solidifying our long-term relationships. So again, *don't knock it till you've tried it*. And keep your mind wide open.

And sometimes your brain just shuts down

There are going to be times when you'll definitely need a lot more than a stress ball to manage your emotions. Distress can get so intense that it activates your brain and your body into overdrive, forcing you into fight-or-flight. Basically, your brain shuts down and your physical body takes over. In these really tough times, using a coloring book is no match for the intensity of your feelings. You'll lose every time.

We need to arm you with the necessary tools to get you back to baseline—decreasing what we professionally call your *emotional arousal*. When you're aroused emotionally, you're quite literally out of your mind. In other words, your body takes over, with your nervous system at the wheel. And since your primal instincts have taken over in these moments, you need to fall back on skills that will activate your parasympathetic nervous system—the part that conserves energy and triggers the body to secrete hormones that decrease blood pressure and heart rate, helping you become more relaxed and present.

One of my favorite foolproof skills to use in these moments is *cold*. Like the 1990s song says, "Ice ice baby!" My office freezer is filled with ice packs for anytime clients or even I need a good chilling out. Using ice on your forehead, neck, or eyelids creates the "dive response." Blood flow rushes to your brain and heart, and your breath and heart rate slow. Extreme cold snaps your mind into the here and now, and helps to slow down your rapid-firing emotions.

If that method doesn't do it for you, diaphragmatic or belly breathing and progressive muscle relaxation, an exercise that involves tensing and relaxing different muscle groups in a methodical way, are both amazing skills to get the parasympathetic system activated. Learning more about these are as easy as Googling them. Get to it!

PUTTING ON MY THERAPIST HAT

Some of you may find yourself triggered, feeling like you're repeating the exact same patterns over and over again. It's as though your judgment simply cannot be accessed. You may get so activated at times, the skills you've practiced simply don't work. This suggests that you may be suffering from trauma. If you're trying really hard and it still feels like these skills aren't working, it's likely not you, it's your trauma, and it may be a good time to look into some specific evidence-based trauma treatment such as EMDR, prolonged exposure, Sensorimotor Psychotherapy, cognitive processing therapy (CPT), present-centered therapy, and Seeking Safety.

Long-Lasting Skills

Right-Now Skills are there for you in the moment, while Long-Lasting Skills help you to fortify the foundation of your new relationship. The more you use both of these skill sets and integrate them into your everyday life, the stronger and more balanced your relationship will become. Right-Now Skills serve the same purpose as a battery, providing you with instant energy to use in the moment. When your regular power supply fails, Long-Lasting Skills help to create a stockpile of extra energy to rely on so you can avoid emergency situations as much as possible. And who doesn't want extra—mind, body, and spirit? The power bank created by practicing Long-Lasting Skills makes you far less susceptible to triggers and cravings, and it allows you to stay in your best self more often and get back to it faster than ever.

It takes a village

Creating human connection is perhaps the most important of all the Long-Lasting Skills. I would say it's not just important, but *fundamental* to your new relationship. And I'm not alone. Research suggests that some of your problems with food correspond to a lack of connection. In one of my favorite studies on connection, rats were isolated in cages and given a choice of plain water or water with heroin. In isolation, these rats chose drugs every single time. When the study was redone, the rats were placed in a park full of fun and community with other rats. This time, the rats chose heroin over water far less frequently than those in isolation.

Isolation can serve as a flourishing petri dish for your dysfunctional relationship with Sugar, negative outlook, and general self-hate. We're pack animals! Connection in community is a necessary part of survival; it's what makes us thrive. And it helps to give us the feeling of kinship, love, joy, and fun that we are endlessly trying to satisfy in the bottom of our ice cream pint, pizza box, or glass of wine. Of course it makes sense that people use substances less when they feel connected and a part of something bigger than themselves.

Brené Brown, a renowned researcher and speaker on vulnerability and shame, and one of my favorite human beings ever to walk the earth, defines connection as "the energy that exists between people when they feel seen, heard, and valued; when they can give and receive without judgment." Making meaningful connections is going to be the saving grace for your new relationship, and Brown's research is largely devoted to this. She's found that connection alleviates shame, which is one of the hallmarks driving you back to your relationship with Sugar. When we feel connected, our shame cannot survive.

There are more ways to connect than I could ever write about. But know this: It most definitely takes a village, and there is a village out there for you to join or create. Connection comes in all different shapes and sizes. There are family and friends, and communities of people who share your struggles, interests, passions, humor, hobbies, or religious and spiritual beliefs. To get even more connected, you can check my website, mollycarmel.com, to see what I'm cultivating for our community.

If you're not connected or connected enough, you have a very solvable problem on your hands. I've never heard anyone complain that they just felt too supported in life, too rooted for, too loved—so get out there and *find your people*. And I beg you to be brave and speedy in your attempt in creating this Long-Lasting Skill. It's a literal lifesaver.

Attitude of gratitude

Being connected also allows us to look at the world beyond the scope of "me, me, me," helping us feel grounded, protected, and supported. This is where connection to something bigger than you comes into play, big-time.

Why do you need a connection to something bigger? If we know something for sure, it's that your relationship with Sugar has made your life—or at least parts of your life—very small. It's impacted your best thinking and decision making, turning it against you. As a result, the voice you're so often listening to is narrow-minded, impulsive, and scared, leaving the solutions to your problems in Sugar's hands.

Creating a connection to something more allows you to expand your mind and change how you look at the world—a skill that's incredibly useful whether or not you're breaking up with Sugar. To quote one of my favorite teachers, Wayne Dyer, "When you change the way you look at things, the things you look at change." Connecting to something bigger helps you to change the way you look at *everything*.

Practicing gratitude is an essential component of this new connection. Research links it to a higher satisfaction with life, helping you to be more optimistic, determined, and able to cope with stressful life events, and to have stronger relationships. It has also shown to be amazing for your physical health—improving sleep and lessening your physical ailments.

On to the *action* of gratitude: My favorite way to practice is by writing a list. Actually, I send a daily text to one of my BFFs, Dria, and she does the same, doubling down on my connection. What a difference it makes! It can put glitter on a gloom-and-doom day pretty quickly. You can keep a gratitude journal, start a group text with your friends, or check out one of my favorite apps, the Five Minute Journal.

Research shows that the practice of prayer or another kind of reflective exercise such as meditation also helps you experience more gratitude throughout your day. Not only that, but prayer has been shown to decrease anxiety and depression, increase immune system functioning, and enhance your self-control.

I'm not necessarily suggesting religion here; praying doesn't have to be to God or any other recognized deity, though of course it can be! It merely needs to be to something outside yourself and your fear—which is usually the feeling that pops up when we close down and isolate. And I most definitely want you to stay connected and grounded in your long-term goals. If you're getting caught up in any connotation or prejudice you may have about this, please try to keep it simple. Your something bigger than you can be the ocean, the moon, the doorknob—it just can't be your fear or your relationship with Sugar.

Remember, when you resign yourself to suffer in silence, you increase your suffering—and your susceptibility to taking Sugar back. Connecting to something bigger is how we stay grounded even in the tough times, and that's what gives us the power to get through things we can't do alone!

Free your mind and the rest will follow

If community is the connection to the external, meditation is the connection to the internal. Beyond a doubt, meditation is one of the single most important practices you can adopt to protect your new relationship with food. My clients who embrace a meditation practice have been the most successful at breaking up with Sugar. Why? There's an overwhelming amount of research illustrating that meditation basically improves everything. It helps regulate behavior, reduce stress, and keep your emotions steady—improving your overall emotional health. It also improves physical health, strengthens the immune system, improves cognitive functioning, aids sleep—the list goes on and on. People who practice meditation have increased awareness of their urges to eat and can create more space between their urges and actions. And the newest research is showing that mindfulness can actually reduce cravings and lead us to eat less. And you know how you turn back to Sugar when you start to obsess about the past or worry about the future? Meditation helps you to stay in the present moment and come back to the moment when your mind wanders off. Essentially, meditation can help us to get *everything* we want in our new relationship!

Feeling stuck on where to start? There are a ton of resources available, many of them free, online, and easily accessible on your phone. You can search for apps such as Headspace, Calm, and Insight Timer. There's also a whole host of free videos on YouTube. Not wanting to head to the internet for your meditation? Easy peasy—focus on one thing in the moment and stay focused on it for five or ten minutes—a sound, a sight, your breath. It's all up to you, and there's no wrong or right way to do it!

I like to move it, move it!

The modern world has locked us in a cage. We sit in cubicles, drive around in cars, and "reward" ourselves with all-day Netflix binges. As with any animal under these constricted circumstances, our physical and mental health suffer. We've forgotten the importance of movement and its counterpart, breath.

Let me be really clear here—I'm not talking about *Biggest Loser*, three-times-a-day, pound-it-until-you-puke exercise. We're getting you into a loving relationship with yourself, and that's no way to live *or* love. Exercising in a compensatory way—like you ate a whole bucket of fried chicken and washed it down with gravy and need to work it off—is a sign of disordered eating. If you check the diagnostic criteria, it looks a whole lot like bulimia.

There really isn't any data that shows that increased exercise *alone* helps you to release weight. It can actually undermine the building of your relationship in small but significant ways, like increasing your appetite, how much you eat, and making you more sedentary after intensely exercising.

So when I'm talking about movement and breath, I'm talking about the loving and healthy kind. I'm talking about your morning walk with your BFF, a long bike ride, taking your favorite Zumba, or exercise-du-jour class, participating in a tennis clinic, dancing to six of your favorite tunes in your bedroom, walking your dog—you get the idea—whatever feels nurturing to your body and soul.

The mental and physical benefits of *moderate* physical activity are undeniable. We feel more energetic and strong. Exercise has been found to decrease stress and depression. And then there are all the physical impacts: reducing the risk of Alzheimer's and dementia, lowering blood pressure, and so much more—which helps us be more skilled at maintaining our loving relationship with food!

And when we move more, we breathe more. You would be amazed at how often you unintentionally trigger your anxiety by not breathing or by breathing through your lungs rather than your diaphragm. With or without exercise, diaphragmatic or deep belly breathing is an excellent way to reduce stress, increase attention, and make you less emotionally reactive. Breathing slowly and deeply is also linked to improved organ functioning, reduced hypertension, and decreased pain. So it's not overstating it to say breathing is the secret to life—and maybe to even reducing your cravings!

You. Need. Joy.

Let's be straight, Sugar's been your great love and your BFF. So it's no wonder you're feeling black-hole lonely! This breakup is hard because you don't believe that anything will taste or feel as good as your beloved Sugar. But remember, your abusive relationship has *hijacked your reward system*, and with the reinforcement of this abuse, your reward system has built up a tolerance. In short, less and less dopamine is released when you're eating food *and* when you're participating in other normally pleasurable activities. Over time, this will pass and your reward system will recover, but to speed up the process, some investigating is in order. Again, don't pull a Betty—keep your mind open and this can be really fun!

We need to bring back your *joy*! Why? When you experience joy, connection, and laughter, your brain releases dopamine, serotonin, and endorphins—chemicals that enhance your feelings of pleasure and block feelings of stress and pain. Practicing joy will help to improve your mood and decrease your feelings of sadness and depression.

Cultivating your creativity is one of the most useful and effective ways to create joy. In our diet drama and despair, not to mention our very busy lives, we may have overlooked creativity. But for many of us, self-hate has suffocated the parts of us that produce gratitude and joy. So practicing creativity is a real must. With the departure of Sugar and Flour, we need to open the door to new things. Practicing creativity helps us to get to know ourselves on a deeper level, fostering self-love. And when there's self-love, Sugar's love doesn't feel nearly as powerful.

Creativity also helps us to break out of our comfort zones. And if we're being honest, our relationship with Sugar has made our comfort zones *super* comfortable—so much so that we don't want to break out of them, *ever*, even though the research tells us that going beyond these zones inoculates us against shame, the feeling that can put us back together with Sugar in three seconds flat.

Trying new things is hard; it can tap into the parts of us that are less than cool and make us vulnerable or feel embarrassed. It's also the skill that can be the jumping-off point for the loving relationship you're creating with yourself. Some of my clients have joined their local musical theater productions and unearthed an unknown and great love for song and dance; others have joined volleyball leagues and discovered how fun group sports can be. I've seen clients take trips abroad and spark a love of culture, take writing classes to reveal their inner author—the list goes on and on. By using food as a skill exclusively, you've stopped doing so many of the things you used to find enjoyable and cut yourself off from learning what you like! When Sugar took over as a hobby, it robbed you of knowing who you are and what brings you joy. Now you have an opportunity—yes, you read that right, an opportunity—to explore who you are and what you love. Isn't that exciting?

Practice makes progress

Depending on what they are, our habits will either make us or break us. We become what we repeatedly do.

—Sean Covey

Routines breed habits; practice makes progress. In a world where people, situations, and events are constantly in flux and Sugar and Flour are trying to bait you at every pass, your habits can provide a sense of control and mastery. They help to fill you with pride, accomplishment, and integrity.

But they require consistent practice—and lots of it. Remember the sixty-six days we're using as a marker for your Sugar breakup? The same marker can be used in creating these new routines and habits with your Right Now and Long-Lasting Skills. So here I am, begging you to make yet *another* commitment to prioritize one or two of these skills—integrate them into your daily routine, and remember that something is always better than nothing. Believe me, you won't be disappointed when your skills help you steer clear of seductive Sugar and demoralizing bingeing and you find yourself moving closer to real joy and freedom.

I Broke Up with Sugar

Josh

Before we broke up, Sugar and I had a deeply complicated love-hate relationship. I loved Sugar because it allowed me to numb my emotions and avoid dealing with the things in my life that weren't working for me. At the same time, I hated Sugar because it caused me to think irrationally and remain morbidly obese, stuck in a vicious cycle of bingeing. My life with Sugar was like living in a fog, with little to no control over my life. I would consume mass quantities of it to shut down uncomfortable feelings and believed I had solved my problem! But you know the story—my urges to eat would return, sometimes within minutes, always stronger than they were before. The cycle of bingeing, depression, and feeling hopeless around food and weight was nonstop and all-encompassing.

My food foundation is based on meal regulation, consistent food choices, and being broken up with Sugar and Flour. I was not a fan of any of these three things when I first instituted them in my life, but once they became more intuitive, I never looked back. Meditation, journaling, calling a supportive friend, and even dunking my head in ice water have all been and continue to be helpful in keeping me broken up for good. Understanding that a slip is simply a tiny blip on the radar has been essential to me. It's about being in it for the long game.

Since breaking up with Sugar, I no longer experience headaches or stomachaches and I don't get tired during the day. My mind is not focused on food, and by eating filling foods that don't contain Sugar, I'm not hungry or craving anything anymore. Before breaking up with Sugar, I was always craving something or thinking about what I would eat next. Now I'm calm, focused, and just generally happier throughout my day. Most important, I'm free and unburdened in a way that allows me to live a life I never knew possible.

I Broke Up with Sugar

Sarah

I always had a love of food, but the correlation between eating and emotions, spirituality, control, and fear started after I experienced a trauma at nine years old. Saying, "I'm fine, I'm fine, I'm fine," became second nature to me. I was living as if my trauma hadn't happened, and instead, whenever I was sad, anxious, or nervous, I ate. I would do anything to get my hands on sugary food. My heart would beat as I approached the cash register with guilt and shame, but also relief that I was moments away from feeling the comfort from the fullness.

My binge eating yo-yoed throughout high school and college. While I lost some weight over the years, I was mentally unhealthy. I had anxiety and very low self-confidence. I continued to eat secretly and "balanced" it out by attempting countless diet programs and using calorie-counting apps.

After I graduated college, I met Molly. Enough was enough. I was overweight, unhappy, guarded, sad, and depressed. The journey really started when I had to face the truth of having an addiction and accepted that bingeing is the one thing in my life that has the power to wreak havoc on everything else. By confronting and radically accepting the problem, I relieved myself of all that built-up guilt and shame. I finally let myself be free and work on skills to overcome it. What has saved me time and again is my food foundations. My foundations are meal regulation, no Sugar or Flour, and keeping a written food log. No matter what, I can count on these patterns to catch me when I'm in difficult situations.

I make smart choices. I accept my disorder instead of using it as an excuse. I have beautiful conversations. I eat for fuel and energy. I move my body for fun instead of as part of a weight-loss goal. The mind-body-soul connection is no joke. For me, it started with letting go of Sugar and Flour, then consciously putting my focus elsewhere: on building my foundation, practicing skills, and putting my new relationship with Sugar and myself as number one on my priority list.

Part 3

Your Breakup

Chapter 10

Scripting Your Farewell Letter

Whether your relationship status is deadbeat loser, compulsive control freak, or full-blown abuser, it's clear that keeping Sugar in your life isn't helping you get any closer to your ideal relationship with food or yourself. Nor are the shaming, limiting Core Beliefs that are attached to it. It's time to say good-bye.

And as much as you may be dying to get over it—to master your food plan and get on with things—you simply can't. You've decided to do it differently this time, right? Every other diet book you've read has put most of its focus on the food. It's glossed over the loss, the beliefs, the future, the critical fact that *this is a relationship*.

Your relationship with Sugar is *deeply personal*. It's a monumental moment, breaking up with this mood-altering substance that gives you comfort, relief, and companionship. It would be very negligent of both of us to assume you don't have to deal with the big feelings that go along with that!

I'm going to walk you through an important exercise: Writing your farewell letter to Sugar. This is about declaring your commitment to yourself and your new relationship. For some of you this may be easy: *My relationship with Sugar is over forever—for good.* One and done. But for many of you, it may not be so simple. It's much more likely that the path will be a little bumpy, with some starts and stops, wavering commitments, urges to return to your abusive relationship, and times when you might even—eek!—invite Sugar back for a quick booty call.

This letter is intended to be your jumping-off point. Motivation waxes and wanes, and while the path to breaking up with Sugar doesn't have to be perfect, your commitment needs to be unwavering. Writing this letter is about decisively stating the facts about your relationship with Sugar and your feelings about it, to make a case for your long-term happiness and goals.

Whatever your breakup is going to look like, you have some feelings to work through. If you're fearful, that's completely normal. Angry and resentful? Totally natural. And given your years of diet drama and trauma, it's probable that you're also experiencing some sadness and hopelessness, too. The healing is in the feeling. Putting pen to paper begins the process of starting your new life, and helps bring clarity to an often bumpy and muddled process.

I'm asking you to call upon your wisest self in scripting a farewell letter to Sugar, a letter in which you air the dirty laundry and speak your truth. No need to panic—there's no rulebook, no right or wrong way to break up. Your exit may be calm, quiet, and solemn—a few words and then Sugar gets the cold shoulder. Or it may be explosive and filled with rage, with you throwing all Sugar's clothes out the apartment window and smashing its TV. They're your feelings and you're entitled to them. How you process them is yours, too. That's all that matters.

I'm just here to help! To get the ball rolling, I made you some fill-in prompts that I've found to be useful for self-reflection. And if that's not fitting the bill, feel free to go off script and create your own. Or start off with a prompt and get lost in your feelings. Again, there is no wrong way. You do you—every way is wonderful.

To make sure that you feel you've honored yourself and this relationship, I'm asking you (again) to schedule some quiet time to reflect and write this letter. You deserve it.

MY FAREWELL LETTER

Dear Sugar,

At the start of our relationship, I thought . . .
* What first drew you to Sugar?
* How did it make you feel in the beginning?
* What problems did Sugar solve for you?

This is how I wished our relationship could be . . .
* Of course you never planned to be here. How do you wish the relationship could have been?

I tried so hard to fix us . . .
* How have you tried to make your relationship seemingly normal?
* Review your list of attempts you've made to diet, cleanse, or eat differently. To make it easier, take a look back to chapter four.

I have been delaying this breakup because I'm scared that . . .
* What fears have gotten in the way of ending this relationship?
* When you imagine your life without Sugar, what feels too hard or difficult?

Our relationship has impacted me in the following ways . . .
* Think about how your life has been impacted by Sugar—the good, the bad, and the ugly.
* What damage has Sugar caused in your life? How has it affected your health, your relationships, your goals, your body, your self-esteem, your hopes, your dreams?
* How has Sugar held you back?

I've been holding on to the following memories . . .
* Memories keep us hooked on the past. What memories are keeping you in the relationship? Is it the idea of birthdays, anniversaries,

and celebrations without Sugar? Nights alone without being soothed by food?

* How would it feel creating new memories without Sugar?
* What are you going to miss the most? Will you miss the rituals? The traditions? The spontaneity? The comfort?

But Sugar, I won't miss . . .

* What *won't* you miss? What are you most looking forward to leaving behind? The feelings of shame and remorse? The harm that Sugar has caused your body? The time you've lost trying to make the relationship work? The deep regret after a binge?

In my new life without you, Sugar, I will . . .

* Explain to Sugar what you need. You are taking your life back and you have every right to ask for what you want. What do you need to move forward? Do you need Sugar to leave you alone as you try my 66-day program and figure out your next steps? How can Sugar show you the respect that you deserve?
* What are you going to do for yourself to help solidify the breakup? Rely on your friends? Get more support? Commit to an open mind? The list can be long or short.
* Anything else you need to say? Make sure you get it down.

Love, Me

When you're done writing, it's time to consider your next steps. This isn't meant to scare you, it's meant to empower you—for the first time you have choices when it comes to this relationship. That's a really good thing. I want you to seriously entertain reading your breakup letter aloud. It's what makes things really *real*—which might feel scary, but ultimately will help you cut the cord. Read it aloud in front of a mirror, to your best friend, or in a place that's sacred to you, like in your backyard, your favorite park—or the Krispy Kreme parking lot. After reading it, perhaps you want to keep it to refer back to when times get tough, or maybe you want to tear it up, burn it, or bury it. This process is yours and yours alone.

I Broke Up with Sugar

Kaitlin

It is impossible to overstate the impact that Molly and breaking up with Sugar have had on my life. Before I found the program, my obsession with dieting (and the inevitable bingeing that accompanied it) ruled my days. When I was "good," I felt limitless and powerful. When I was "bad," I hid from the world, certain I was sick, devoid of willpower, and unworthy of love. My life felt like a house of cards; regardless of what I accomplished at work or otherwise, my relationship with food reinforced that I was a failure. Feeling dejected by years of therapy that led to zero relief, by my late twenties it felt like the writing was on the wall: I was destined to remain this way forever.

By the time I found Molly, I was so desperate and defeated that I barely balked when she told me I had to give up Sugar, Flour, and dieting. At that point, the problem was so much bigger than weight. All I wanted was to wake up and not feel like I had hurt myself for the thousandth time. Still, as a natural-born skeptic who had tried and failed to "get better" more times than I can count, I figured this would be just another attempt.

To my surprise, once I began adhering to the food guidelines, I found immediate relief. For the first time in my life, I felt free: free from the fear that I was going to binge and free from the constant shame I felt from hiding my secret. After a lifetime of closely counting calories and avoiding carbs and fat, I now love what I eat. The meal plan leaves me satisfied and nourished and makes eating out (an activity I used to dread) a pleasant experience. For the first time in my life, I'm treating my body—a body that has treated me superbly well, despite not getting that same respect—the way it deserves to be treated.

No longer preoccupied by an endless spiral of shame, I suddenly see textures and colors I only imagined before, and have enough space in my mind and heart to let them in. I would break up with Sugar a thousand times for the freedom that I've gained.

I Broke Up with Sugar

Jeannine

My relationship with food prior to the breakup was full of highs and lows, bumps and grooves, and very little smooth riding. There was no control; food was all excitement and impulse. I used it to keep my adrenaline pumping, yet, looking back now, I realize I was just running on fumes.

All my past attempts to diet were focused on the actual food I was eating, not the core reasons I was consuming certain foods and how it was impacting my life. Once I understood how Sugar and Flour impacted my overall health, not just my weight, well, it just clicked! Sugar was unknowingly in my foods all the time, and I had no idea that I was in such an unhealthy relationship with it!

With Sugar and Flour out of my life, there are so many things I focus on now. Food is no longer the only thing. I'm aware of how my body is feeling, and I use food as fuel and energy to live instead of as a reward or a way to soothe. I no longer feel bloated all the time—totally surreal! I've learned to practice meditation, which helps me be present and notice my behaviors, reactions, impulses, and stress levels. I've gained clarity on who I am and what my physical and emotional needs are. I surround myself with people who acknowledge and support my choices and goals—those I can learn from and continue to be challenged by, who appreciate the person I am as I evolve to be more than I thought I could be.

I now feel like I have control over what's going on my plate and am confident enough about it to communicate with those preparing the food (even if it is myself sometimes!). Confidence—now, that's a win to celebrate, too! It feels amazing at the end of the day to realize all the good choices I made during the day, all the celebrated wins. It helps me go to bed and fall asleep quickly and peacefully, and I wake up each morning well rested. Coming off a lifestyle of insomnia, it's such a great feeling to be refreshed after a night of good sleep.

Finally, I learned I can be healthy. I learned what healthy *feels like*. I learned that it's possible, no matter what phase, stage, or time period we are going through in life. I now understand and believe that it's sustainable for my lifestyle. I now believe in myself.

Chapter 11

Purgatory: Hold Up.
What Did I Just Do?!

B reakup letter written and read, maybe even buried or burned . . .
Check! Your feelings about that? Unknown.

You may be feeling a sense of lightness and relief because you've finally figured that Sugar is the root of much of the angst and havoc in
your life. Or you may be in a daze, telling yourself that none of this is a
big deal. You may be curled up in a ball on the floor, hysterically crying,
wondering what the eff you just did by breaking up with the great love
of your life. Or you may be having all the feels. Put on your wetsuit; the
waves of feelings are coming.

When you start to focus on your recovery, it's also common for the
feelings that you've been eating and denying to rise up, often erupting
like a volcano: betrayal, anger, fear, sadness, grief. And I'm with you—
when I first decided to break up with Sugar, I felt a tsunami of emotions. I was horrified, fearful, depressed, and filled to the brim with
rage. I *literally* spent nights screaming and crying on my kitchen floor.

First things first: *This is completely and totally normal.* You've been
in this relationship for years—it's come to define your experience of the
world! Saying good-bye isn't easy—just ask every single tragic love
song, poem of passion, heartbroken meme, and rom-com.

Without question, there will be some serious pushback from Sugar
coming your way, especially given all the warm memories that have
burrowed into your brain over the years. The state you're in may feel a

little like purgatory, the waiting place between heaven and hell. I'm going to help you move past it, and the only way is straight through. So let's get moving!

I'm sure this isn't your first time dealing with feelings like these. It may be the first time you're dealing with them without numbing and pushing them down with your beloved Sugar. But still, it's likely you have *some* experience here. Don't underestimate yourself—if you find yourself questioning, judging, or being fearful of your emotional reactions, think about other times in your life when you've lost something or someone important. When someone you loved passed away, a partner broke up with you, or you lost a job, didn't you feel pain? Didn't you have some reaction? *Loss is loss.* And losing your relationship with Sugar is a biggie. That's what you're experiencing here—straight-up loss. Which comes with a whole host of feelings that we're going to use this chapter to address and help to soften the blow.

I know firsthand how difficult this breakup is, but I also know that the immense pain of this loss is truly the entrance fee to the soul-expanding freedom on your horizon.

YOU'RE NOT GOING CRAZY. YOU'RE *GRIEVING*.

Headline: Your feelings are normal, albeit totally uncomfortable. Your skin may feel like it's crawling or too tight, the echo of "What did I do?" may be on repeat in your head, or maybe you're just frozen with fear. No matter what you're experiencing, there's no need to worry. You're not going crazy. Actually, you're exactly where you need to be.

This, my friends, is grieving. And it's just a phase. Phew!

Grieving is an inevitable part of this journey. You may be thinking, *Grief? Seriously? Nobody died!* Grief is commonly defined as "a natural reaction to significant emotional loss of any kind" or the experience of having "conflicting feelings caused by the end of or a change in a familiar pattern of behavior." Sound familiar? Let's get real: We grieve whenever we experience a significant loss. And your relationship with Sugar was *significant*, to say the least.

We all grieve differently; it's a very personal process. I'm not going to tell you what your grief *will* or *should* look like. But there's a lot we can learn from our buddies science and research to help you move through it, and keep focused on your path to freedom.

The late psychiatrist Elisabeth Kübler-Ross is the go-to for all things bereavement. In her renowned work with terminally ill patients, she began to notice a common theme in the emotions experienced through this process. She created a groundbreaking model that identifies five stages of grief: denial, anger, bargaining, depression, and acceptance. These feelings can be experienced in any order, without any sort of timeline. We can begin our process in acceptance, then move to anger or bargaining later on. All of these emotions are completely normal and are to be expected—though there's no telling when and where they'll show up, or even if they will at all.

Feelings are wonderful indicators and information grabbers. They let us know when something is wrong, when something is right, when we need to be cautious and wary. They often compel us to action. And while they are very savvy, they're not exactly facts, especially when you're grieving. During this process, I need you to be very careful about what you're feeling and thinking, most particularly about the *actual truth* of your thoughts and the cost of acting upon them. As I've told you before, action is a thousand times more potent than thought. Some of the feelings you're going to experience may make you idealize Sugar and want to hightail it back to your old relationship faster than you can say "doughnut." And we definitely do-nut want that.

Is any of this fair? Nope. But is it true? Yup. So let's file this under Knowledge Is Power. We're going to review the stages of grief, so you can feel informed and empowered in your process. You're not alone or overreacting. You got this, and as always, I've got your back.

ALL THE FEELS
Denial

Do you know those moments in life when you're hit with an incredibly overwhelming truth? Your first thought is *There's no way this is happening*. It's like we throw a blanket over our heads so we don't have to see what's right in front of us. It's a form of self-preservation called *denial*.

We rely on our ability to deny when we're faced with a reality that feels too distressing or painful to accept. It's a natural coping mechanism. It's actually very useful. Why? It allows us to continue functioning in the "comfort" to which we have become accustomed.

Why is it so hard to wrap your head and your heart around the idea that your relationship with Sugar was abusive and is now over? Jack Nicholson wasn't kidding when he said in *A Few Good Men*, "You can't handle the truth!" He's right. Your brain is designed to help you avoid pain. The reason you wouldn't step into moving traffic is the same reason you're having a hard time accepting this breakup. When the pain receptor is triggered, your brain is immediately cued to do what's necessary to shut it down.

If you're in denial about the extent to which Sugar rules your life or you find yourself feeling numb to this new reality, I get it. It's hard to let it sink in. If you're chilling in Camp Denial, why don't you ask it, "Denial, what exactly are you trying to protect me from?" Chances are it's scared of a future without Sugar. And while a future sans-Sugar *is* scary, the future trapped in its grip may be even more frightening. Denial about the *real* problem is slowing down your process—in many cases to an absolute crawl. And that's the real purgatory.

Anger

In my experience, anger is the poster child of the grieving process. Hear me loud and clear: Anger, or ANGERRRRRRR, as it's more commonly experienced, is normal, and it abounds when we're dealing with loss. It's so often powered by a sense of injustice: *Why the heck do I have to have this problem? It isn't fair that I have to give up Sugar and Sally doesn't! This is such a joke. Nothing is ever going to be as good as Sugar! Why am I doing this?*

And with food it can be especially unfair—it's everywhere, provoking you at every turn. If it was heroin you were breaking up with, you wouldn't have to worry about opening Instagram and seeing successful, happy people shooting up in public. With Sugar we see CEOs, models, and movie stars eating and enjoying it all the time, seemingly with ease. Having to admit that we can't do the same is a hard pill to swallow.

And it can spark wrath at any minute of the day. It's *beyond* unfair, and it can make us feel willful and resistant to accept that Sugar can't be in our lives.

Anger namaste: The anger in me honors the anger in you. I hear your anger and I can tell you, I've been there, too. This was my primary emotion when I was breaking up with Sugar. I was a rage machine. The sense of injustice you feel is accurate—so let that anger out. And while it's totally an option to run down the street screaming and biting the heads off each and every person who crosses your path, I don't really advise it. It makes much more sense to punch a pillow, take a kickboxing class, or scream the tiles off your bathroom walls. Acting out the anger in inappropriate ways will only give you more problems to deal with, and your breakup already provides plenty of issues to solve.

Bargaining

Ahh, the bargaining stage. So aptly described as the *what-if* and *if-only* stage. This is when you are most vulnerable to reexposing yourself to Sugar's toxic glow, so let's put on some extra sunscreen.

Bargaining can really do a number on your staunch decision to break up with Sugar. You're longing to return to the way things were in hopes that this was all just a really, really bad dream. Boy, do I get it. But remember, the real bad dream is actually your destructive relationship with Sugar.

In bargaining, you start to rationalize your relationship, or as you know I love to call it, rational-lies. Your mind reverts to believing that maybe, just maybe you can make things work (*you can't*); maybe it wasn't so bad after all (*it was*). You try to negotiate the price of this breakup.

You say things like: *I'll give up Sugar if I can just have pumpkin pie at Thanksgiving. I'll exercise three times a day if I can just have my sweet at night. I won't eat Sugar when I'm alone, but when I'm out to dinner I'll eat what I want. I don't think Sugar is the problem; it's definitely salt.* We can drive ourselves batty with all the arguments we can come up with in this stage, putting the delusions of the past on repeat and fantasizing about how to outsmart the system. It's safe to presume that we've hit the great wall between ourselves and full acceptance.

A loving warning: While this is totally a normal part of the grieving process, you need to make sure that you keep the bargaining as thoughts, not behaviors. Acting on bargaining can shove you right back into the arms of Sugar.

Depression

Tears, darkness, that empty pit in our stomachs. DE-PRES-SION. Depression often rides with his pals, loneliness, fear, anxiety, and shame. Like the classic movie scene: You're flipping through old photographs, overwhelmed with sadness at what you've lost and what you're missing, and the terror that you'll never, ever love like this again rising inside. Sound familiar? I can remember literally crying at the idea of never having dark chocolate cake again. And I don't even like dark chocolate.

Of course your breakup with Sugar feels sad and scary, like you're discarding the life you know and plunging into uncharted territory. It can be terrifying, lonely making, and guilt producing.

Take caution. As with all these states, it is natural to feel some intense emotions. And while for many of us, our natural tendency is to retreat into isolation when we're down, that reaction puts Miracle-Gro on your already flourishing sadness. Perhaps consider doing the exact opposite: Connect with another person, someone you trust. You know how strongly I (and the research) feel about connection helping you to heal. This is *the* moment to "plug in" and reach out for support, professional or personal.

Acceptance

Acceptance may feel impossible—like a fake stage I included to make you feel better and less hopeless about your breakup. Fear not, it's real—and more important, it's where you will spend the majority of your life after you've gone through the initial stages of grief. #pinkyswear

This is when you stop fighting reality. You may not realize that's what you're doing, but it is. And as it turns out, when we end the struggle, we have less suffering and more serenity. Hard to believe, yet completely true. Research characterizes acceptance as "the experience of inner peace and tranquility that comes with letting go of a struggle to regain what is lost or being taken away." Um . . . yes, please!

In acceptance, we have surrendered the idea of "what was" to face and hopefully embrace the idea of "what is." Often, we don't necessarily love this reality, but we have come to peaceful terms with it. We have accepted our vulnerabilities and susceptibilities to Sugar, the abuse and the time we have lost to the relationship. We're done second-guessing the breakup. It's not to say that we don't think about Sugar or even experience a yearning for the old times—of course we do! But in acceptance, we have a greater ability to detach from these thoughts, especially in light of the amazing life that lies ahead.

Please be gentle. While acceptance may be the end goal, we don't arrive here overnight. Give yourself a minute.

THE RITE OF PASSAGE

I need you to experience this loss, not shy away from it. And we don't need to reinvent the wheel here. Every spiritual and religious tradition honors grief through ritual, and so shall you. Research shows that people who mourn with rituals experience decreased levels of grief and increased feelings of control after a loss. And—good for us—the effects hold true regardless of whether someone believed the rituals would actually be effective. So while doing rituals may seem hokey, they work anyway!

I've compiled a bunch of rituals below. Don't get hung up on picking the "perfect" one or not knowing exactly what to choose. Try a few on for size. Research shows that the *type* of ritual you choose is not important; the key is simply to do it. And if these aren't jibing with you, please get creative and try your own ideas! It's your relationship to grieve—your unique rituals help honor your feelings about Sugar and make you feel more in control while saying good-bye to your old life.

> **Make a grief box.** Create an actual container for your grief. The box will hold all your written thoughts and feelings while you are

breaking up with Sugar. Whatever comes to you, whenever it comes, jot it down on a piece of paper and throw it inside. This box acts as your sacred space for all your grief associated with this loss.

Have a candlelight vigil. Light a special candle, used only for this ritual, at a specific time of day or week or just when the grief feels especially poignant.

Create a healing space. Find a place outdoors. Plant a seed and mark the location. This will be your healing place that you can go to grieve and honor the breakup.

Dance it out. Create a dance that expresses your feelings about your breakup with Sugar.

Write poetry. Working on poetry—or any creative writing—that embodies your state of grief can help you let it out.

Party on. Have a (Sugar-free) breakup party with loved ones that celebrates your breakup with Sugar.

Sage your home. Use sage to cleanse your apartment or house post-breakup. This is a ceremonial gesture used in many spiritual practices to symbolize healing and purity.

IT MORE THAN EMOTIONAL. IT'S CHEMICAL.

Ending your relationship with Sugar will come with physical fallout, too. You're breaking up with a substance, not a person. When you have a dependency on a substance and stop consuming it, there are aftereffects. Sugar is no different from other substances that impact your dopamine and reward system—stopping results in withdrawal symptoms. So if you're feeling tired, sad, or irritable, or have headaches, muscle aches, an upset stomach, sleep problems, or intense cravings, you're not going crazy; you're experiencing Sugar detox.

If you've ever let go of another substance, like cigarettes or alcohol (or know someone who has), you know how agonizing these feelings can be. And while your bread and ice cream withdrawal symptoms may not be as intense as delirium tremens, it can feel that way! Physical withdrawal from Sugar has been reported to last from two days to two weeks. During this time, your endocrine and nervous systems are hard at work, getting used to receiving less glucose than they're accustomed to. And that would make anyone feel out of sorts. And remember, the symptoms become less intense the longer you go without Sugar!

As with dealing with your feelings of grief, I want you to have some action items to hold on to while your body is settling into this new Sugar-free state. A quick reminder: *Do not give in and go back to Sugar. Even though it may feel like the only solution to this pain, it only extends your detox.* I know you know that, but one more reminder never hurts.

What to do while you're waiting out withdrawal:

Connection counts. Let your people know you're struggling and ask for some support.

Create a safe space. Make sure you *don't* have your favorite Sugar and Flour foods easily available to you, and make sure you *do* have your favorite new foods on hand.

Keep it simple. This isn't the week to start a new hobby, travel to a new country, or go on a first date. Putting unnecessary challenges on the agenda makes a hard time even harder. And there's no need for that!

Practice self-care. Get a whole lot of rest (withdrawal can make you feel like a hibernating bear!), drink lots of water, take your medications on time, and eat at your normal mealtimes. Throw yourself a little love!

Rely on your skills. Your Right-Now Skills were made for this moment! Listen to music, take the dog to the park, or try some ice packs to calm down during this time.

Remember, it all passes—the good, the bad, the grief, the withdrawal. You'll get through it, and you'll be stronger and in better shape for the very best relationship with food and yourself.

I Broke Up with Sugar

Leah

My struggles with weight go back to my early twenties when I was in college. There, I was surrounded by women who were obsessed with their looks, their weight, and their eating habits. They ate fat-free pretzels, ate only bagels for lunch, and walked the three-mile "loop" at all hours of the day. Being immersed in this odd culture helped me avoid gaining the classic Freshman Fifteen, but I knew it wasn't healthy or sustainable.

After college, I got a job working as an instructor with adjudicated youth in an outdoor setting. Eating Dairy Queen Blizzards or McDonald's Big Macs with french fries was a way to handle the mix of emotions that inevitably came up spending so much time with tough kids in a remote environment. As my career developed, I took with me the lessons I had learned from working with those youth, along with my eating habits. Sedentary jobs and more access to food created negative consequences of my eating that caught up with me quickly. For the first time in my memory, I was at a weight that didn't feel healthy to me. I dove into diets. While I lost some weight at first, I always felt like the diets failed to address some key emotional element to my eating. After thirteen years of an on again, off again relationship with Weight Watchers, I met Molly.

I learned about how our brains respond to Sugar and Flour the same way they do cocaine. This was staggering information but absolutely made sense to me! I reflected on my work as a therapist. When talking with clients who had experience with addiction, I would often say that while I am not a drug addict or alcoholic, I never met a piece of chocolate that I didn't like. I'm that person who can't keep a bowl of M&M's in my office because I will eat them all in one day. Once I taste a cupcake with buttercream frosting, there is no going back, and I'll eat more if they are available. So as Molly was describing the connection between Sugar and our brains, it completely resonated with me.

But I was terrified. Sure, I wanted to make changes so that I would be healthier, but in my heart of hearts I also dreaded making the commitment to give up things I thought I loved. I agreed to her offer, telling myself it was only for sixty-six days. I went home and cleaned out my fridge and cabinets, went shopping, and began the journey. While I was feeling empowered, I also quickly encountered a flood of feelings of grief and loss. I was mad that someone was telling me I couldn't eat Flour. I was irritated that I had to read food labels and not buy things that had Sugar in the first four ingredients. I was annoyed with our food industry for putting Sugar into everything in the grocery store. Who knew bacon had Sugar in it?!

Once I hit the sixty-six-day mark, I felt proud of myself. I saw a difference on the scale, and more important, I felt so much better. I was no longer going through my usual emotional swings. And since I wasn't eating Sugar, there wasn't anything to be hard on myself about. Now here I am, almost four years later and still at it. Thankfully, Molly has been by my side since day one. She reminds me to be gentle with myself and to not be too rigid. Her use of the harm-reduction model has taught me that I can do my best, even in the toughest situations. I no longer let slip-ups derail all the good intentions I have for myself. Molly asks me questions that make me curious about my choices instead of shaming what I've done. I'm now so much more educated and aware of how the choices I make surrounding food have a much larger impact on my life than I previously understood. What's more, I've finally found the link between emotional eating and weight loss that was missing for me from other programs. I'm so grateful to Molly for introducing me to this journey and supporting me along the way.

Chapter 12

Finding Love Again:
It's Closer Than You Know

All this talk about how Sugar and Flour have negatively affected your life—the relationship status, the good-bye letter, the grief—can make you forget there's actually an upside to this whole breakup process!

We are not at a dead end, my friends. Far from it, in fact: We are at a turning point. This is not the end of your life; it's your new and exciting beginning. The road ahead might be unknown, but *you* are in the driver's seat! And I'm here to be your copilot and guide you—you're not traveling that road alone.

So enough of all the Debbie Downer stuff. Let's step into the light that is your solution. Let's talk about the new, better, brighter, more hopeful life that's on the other side of this heartbreak. Because *you are going to find love again.* I know it may feel impossible, but I promise you deep, real, lasting love with food and with yourself is on its way.

And this time, your relationships are going to Love. You. Back.

TAKING BACK YOUR POWER

The unhealthy relationship you've had with Sugar has been your normal for what may feel like forever, so of course it's hard to remember what a healthy relationship with food looks like, or to believe such a thing is even possible. Sugar has taken your power from you, but this chapter is going to start to reverse that.

I need us to agree on one thing first, though. You are not a victim. You are not weak. You are not lazy. Sugar and Flour have caused you to believe that, but the reclamation of your power begins right now. *You. Have. Choices.* And we're going to replace your perceived weakness with real strength, trade your shame for dignity, and exchange your laziness for power. It's all a choice, and we're going to create a new normal instead of letting your very broken status quo continue. It's time to take your power back, so you can focus on the loving relationship you deserve.

THE BROKEN COMPASS

Your value system with food has been corrupted. Despite having solid values, you've behaved toward food in a way that has not been supportive of them. Waking up and solemnly swearing that today is different, then breaking that oath with Sugar by ten a.m. has destroyed your faith in yourself. You've probably never thought to extend your value system to your food. If you did, you might find that your value system in your relationship with Sugar is rooted in immediacy, fear, and shame. That needs to change immediately.

Every relationship has values that guide it. Values are principles or judgments that help you recognize what is important and meaningful. These values help to navigate your course—what to say yes to, what to say no to, what you want, and what you need. Your values are like a compass—they help to guide you toward your true north. Right now, thanks to Sugar, you're struggling with a broken compass, which makes it hard to be faithful to your values.

But not to worry, this is a problem to be solved!

The first thing we need to do is establish a set of values for you—guiding principles that can help you to manage the problems and issues that arise in your life. Then we need to understand your why, which is your motivation for repairing this relationship, getting up in the morning, doing difficult things, and working so earnestly at building this beautiful life. Knowing your why will help you repair your compass and feel confident about the direction in which you are moving.

You may have dismissed these kinds of ideas in the past, thought them unimportant or unnecessary, even in such an essential area of your life. But you need a compass or a North Star to guide you or you will be forever lost. Your Guiding Values and your why will help guide you through the foggiest skies and the rockiest mountains, allowing you to reach new heights with ease.

Guiding Values: Your true north

Your Guiding Values are your true north—they help to orient you and to point you in the direction that will let you stay true to yourself. They are there when the going gets tough and you don't know what to do. They are there when the going gets *amazing* and you don't know what to do.

Creating Guiding Values is a principle of acceptance and commitment therapy (ACT). ACT is an evidence-based therapy centered on acting in accordance with your values, and one that has been shown to be effective in both addiction recovery *and* weight loss. Research tells us that when people determine their values and behave consistently with them, they are less impulsive, more able to tolerate pain, and experience less discomfort. Sound like what you need in this new relationship? Let's get started!

What's the first step in establishing your Guiding Values? Start by answering these questions:

* How do I want to feel in my new life?
* What is important to me?
* How do I want to feel in my new relationship with food?
* How do I want to feel in my new relationship with myself?

When you know how you want to feel—and what you value in these areas—figuring out what to do to feel this way will be easy peasy.

Below you will find a list of the most common Guiding Values. Look through them and see what resonates, then choose three that will be the bedrock of your relationship foundation.

If there's something on the list that you're not seeing, then add it! I've seen people add Divinity, Woot!, Sunshine, Mac (my old dog who I sometimes use as my Guiding Value). The value list is endless, and the most important point is that these values are yours, so they need to be right on the mark. And know that you're going to change through this relationship process—sometimes very quickly—and with that your values might, too, so stay flexible.

COMMON GUIDING VALUES

Adventure	Freedom	Optimism
Assertiveness	Fulfillment	Passion
Authenticity	Fun	Peace
Balance	Gratitude	Perseverance
Clarity	Growth	Respect
Compassion	Happiness	Security
Connection	Health	Self-respect
Consistency	Honesty	Service
Courage	Humility	Stability
Creativity	Humor	Strength
Dependability	Independence	Success
Discipline	Integrity	Supportiveness
Enthusiasm	Joy	Sustainability
Evolution	Kindness	Trust
Fairness	Love	Truth
Faith	Loyalty	Uniqueness
Family	Mindfulness	Vulnerability
Flexibility	Openness	Wisdom

Having these Guiding Values will make your relationship with food so much easier and clearer. One of my clients, Amanda, was starting to worry about her night-eating habits during her Sugar breakup. She shared that she had overeaten four nights of the week. It certainly wasn't as harmful as her past episodes, which were full of Sugar and Flour. She wasn't sure if that accounted for a binge, if this was something she should worry about. When she sought my opinion about her predicament, I simply asked her about her values and if the decision to eat at night brought her closer to them. She shared that her Guiding Values were Freedom, Adventure, and Creativity.

After some chatting, she recognized that her night eating was taking her further from her values. It most definitely made her feel hindered the next day, with bloat and disappointment, which impacted her sense of freedom. Her weight had started to rise, which impacted her capacity for adventure, and she was obsessing about night eating, which got in the way of her creativity. She started to exercise her skills in earnest and was able to eventually eliminate the night eating, taking it down to levels that were far more aligned with her values, without doing much harm to her long-term relationship with food.

When decisions feel confusing and you're not sure if Sugar is stealthily knocking at the door, you can always ask yourself, "Does this decision bring me closer to my Guiding Values?" And your next course of action will be clear as a bell.

YOUR WHY: THE LIGHT AT THE END OF THE TUNNEL

While this breakup comes with lots of amazingness, you will undoubtedly also go through some hard times, when you will lose your way and you'll want to turn back the clock to the way things used to be. Hear me loud and clear: There is nothing worth fighting for more than this.

With your Guiding Values identified, it's now time to create a crystal clear reasoning of why you are moving on from your destructive relationship with Sugar and Flour into this big and beautiful life you're pursuing. In your past flings with diets and nutrition plans, you were probably working off of *what* to do and *how* to do it, with no clear vision of *why* you were doing it in the first place.

Nietzsche said it best: "He who has a Why to live for can bear almost any How." The *why* component of your new relationship is truly the crucial driving force. So for this thing to work long term, your why needs to be deeply instilled in your foundation—mind, body, and soul.

Your brain's limbic system explains why your why is so important. The limbic system is the section of your brain that processes emotions and feelings. Without it we would be completely apathetic, lacking all motivation to do anything. It's also the area of the brain associated with learning and memory. Obviously, the limbic system is essential when you're considering changing a behavior. Or creating a new relationship.

Here are some examples of my client's whys: I want to feel hopeful, confident, loved, healthy/I want to have the lead role and not a supporting one/I want to be me/I want to be vital and mobile/I want to be healthier, be able to play sports, sit in an airplane seat/I want to be healthier for my kids/I want to heal this bingeing and restricting relationship I have with food/I want to manage my diabetes and lower my blood sugar. . . . The list goes on and on.

Your why is *so* important and often overlooked in traditional "destination dieting"—where you're dieting to reach a number on a scale, which inevitably ends in failure. Your why may be unclear; it may not have occurred to you what motivated you to pick up this book in the first place. If you haven't taken the time to consider your why, I need you to make some time to reflect on that before you turn to the next chapter. If you're thinking, *I just want to lose weight. I want to look good for my sister's wedding. I want to wear a size 10*, try to dig a bit deeper. Those are all filed under destination dieting—they all come with expiration dates, which makes a long-term relationship impossible. Consider your why an opportunity to get in touch with your deeper feelings, emotions, and internal desires.

After you've given it some thought, write down your Why—your top three motivators for cutting Sugar and Flour out of your life. Keep them handy—my clients have put them into their phones as a daily reminder, posted them on their fridge, and shared them with friends. The closer you are to your whys, the more seamless it will feel to create this new relationship with food and yourself. Along with your Guiding Values, these are going to be the driving force to keep you on your path to your beautiful, bold, bright relationship.

I Broke Up with Sugar

Stevie

For a long time, I've known that I use food as my drug. I understood that I did not experience hunger or relate to food in the same way others do, but I also felt like I was making excuses for myself for not being strong enough to stay on a diet. I was sinking in all my self-hate and perceived failure, still chasing the next fix, diet, or binge.

I walked into Molly's clinic feeling shattered and brokenhearted. I was moving through the world with a cloud of sadness hanging over me, pushing myself through my pain, shame, and exhaustion with every bit of energy I could muster. I was so depleted and foggy it was hard to even get out of bed.

Working with Molly empowered me with the science, the evidence, and most important, the emotional and spiritual support to identify my abusive relationship with Sugar and Flour and fully own that I am a food addict. It's been so liberating to me! I understand now that no diet will work for me in the long run, but creating a new relationship with food and with myself *will*.

I am not weak or a failure—I have an addiction and need to heal toward my solution. For me, that is learning to manage my life and my feelings without turning to Sugar as my skill and crutch.

Since breaking up with Sugar, Flour, and dieting, I've begun to move off the sidelines of my life to be more fully alive, reconnect with myself, and take more risks. I actually feel good about myself—and that feeling is motivating and uplifting. It's one of hope and gratitude.

Today, I practice a new way of living. My choice is no longer perfection or bust. I don't have to run away or look for a quick-fix magical solution, and I don't have to beat myself up anymore if I struggle. Instead, I brush myself off and get right back to my plan. I stay committed to myself and my integrity, my new relationship with food and myself. Because my life is now about hope, opportunity, love, kindness, and being really present in my life. It's about my twenty-year-old daughter turning to me and saying, "Mom, since Molly, you are a joy," and so for me, this new life is everything.

Part 4

Your Happily Ever After

Chapter 13

Getting to Gray:
How to Stay the Course

You know all too well what it's like to start a diet and end a diet. You know the anticipation and optimism that you wake up with on day one, the frustrating grunt work of day four, and the explosive breakup on day seven. I'd bet that once or twice you were going strong, and then, seemingly out of nowhere, something happened. Things got rough. You may have had a second when you fantasized about what life was like with Sugar—the comfort, the feel-good moments, the crazy highs—and forgot all the bad memories: the sleepless nights, the self-loathing, the physical and emotional discomfort. And in that moment, your greatest ex-love showed up on your porch, roses in hand, serenading you with love songs.

And just like that, you and Sugar were an item again, picking up the relationship right where you left off—with the bags of cookies, dozens of doughnuts, pounds of pasta. Off to the races until the next time you hit a shame-filled, demoralizing rock bottom. Go big or go home, right? *Not anymore.* If you do what you've always done, you'll get what you've always gotten—and we're in the create-a-new-relationship game now. We need to find a different and more effective solution for dealing with your awful ex.

Your mentality about food and your ability to be flexible have been warped. You've become more like a light switch than a dimmer—you're either on or you're off. You're either right or you're wrong. You're either good or you're bad. This black-and-white thinking—which diets are notorious for—has feuled the demise of your relationship with food.

Diets don't provide you any alternatives to these polarized positions. There's no manual to help you when you don't want to do what you know you're supposed to do, when you're feeling too tired, too defiant, when you're in situations where you just can't follow the plan. And, as we well know by now, relationships get tricky. If you're going to create a relationship that stands the test of time, you're going to need some guidelines so that you have alternatives to this black-or-white perfectionism trap that dieting has caught you in.

The on- or off-the-diet mentality causes some of the greatest harm to your spirit, with the starting and stopping over and over (and over!) reinforcing the idea that you just can't do it. It gets demoralizing real quick. You think, *Maybe there's something wrong with me. Maybe I'm just not capable of this.*

These feelings are a function of the diets, not you. You've been set up for failure, which attracts you to other short-term diets that inevitably fail you, because you've never been taught to live in the gray area of your relationship with food. Until now.

NO MORE SLASHING TIRES

One of the cornerstones of your negative relationship with food lies in your commitment to perfectionism. Everything is either going great, or everything is a disaster. We often believe that perfectionism brings us closer to our goals by pushing us harder and forcing us to demand more of ourselves. And sometimes this is the case. But after treating thousands of perfectionists, I see that it causes far more harm than good. It's really hard to berate yourself into wellness. When you're not allowed to make a mistake, you're painting an unrealistic picture of reality, one that's absolutely impossible to live in. *I've got this; I'm going to be perfect. No slips. Period.* Then, when life gets lifey, as it always does, instead of recognizing a misstep, calling it out, course-correcting, and moving on mindfully, you throw a tantrum and quit. *Screw it! I took a bite, might as well have the whole piece . . . well, actually, the whole pie!*

The fancy psychological term for this is the *abstinence violation effect* (AVE): *This is useless, I just can't do it, there's no use in me even trying. I'M DONE.* The AVE is the national anthem of relapse—and it is truly what gets us stuck in the gruesome cycle of continual failure.

Let's get real: If you behaved with the abstinence violation effect in *any* relationship in your life, it, too, would fail. You don't have a hard day at work, flip the desk, and quit your job. You don't have a random fight with your best friend, call it quits on the relationship, and disown her. And yet, *with food, that's exactly what you do.*

Using the abstinence violation effect to guide you in relationships is like getting a flat tire on your car, and instead of fixing the tire or asking for help, you get out of the car, slash all four tires, torch the car, and leave it on the highway! It's a completely unmanageable way to live, and certainly not one that is going to get you into a loving and healthy relationship . . . with yourself, with food, or with anyone.

The solution to this dilemma is tricky. Because it's not black or white. It's gray. And gray is where we need to live in the relationship game. Buckle up—we're moving into uncharted territory, but it's going to free you from this cycle.

So we know that, on the one hand, absolute perfection is not going to be your stand-alone solution, as much as you may wish for that to be the case. You've tried that. Slips are bound to happen. But allowing for slips all the time isn't a long-term solution, either. Constantly backsliding is part of what got you into this mess to begin with, and it doesn't allow you to nurture a healthy relationship. It makes change and growth impossible, which is exactly why we are here.

If total perfection isn't the answer, and unchecked slipups aren't the answer, what *is* the answer? We need a whole new way to manage your mistakes. And guess what? I have one for you! Dr. Marsha Linehan, creator of my favorite therapy ever, DBT, calls this concept *dialectical abstinence*. I like to call it the *Anti-Perfection Plan*. The Anti-Perfection Plan says: *The answer is never the opposite, but rather the balance.* And let's be honest, balance is not our strong suit—*yet*.

It's not balance, exactly. I don't want you pursuing perfection 50 percent of the time and then slipping the other 50 percent of the time.

Those numbers won't sustain the relationship of your dreams. I need you to strive for mostly perfection and make a commitment to get right back on the proverbial horse when slips do happen. If I had to put numbers on that, it would look like you're mostly adherent, rocking and rolling about 85 percent of the time and having *unplanned* slips the other 15 percent. Here's how we're going to get there:

Go for the Gold!

When your experience has been mostly serious diet drama and trauma, starting your day with humble optimism is a big ask. That's because many of you are accustomed to waking up in the morning with a shrug of your shoulders, complacent with the idea that you're going to behave like you have every other day of your life—that is, letting yourself down and turning to Sugar. This is a behavior that needs to stop immediately—like, yesterday. Starting your day with that kind of resignation is like an Olympian saying they are going to "go for the bronze" before a big event. You and I both know that aiming for a bronze means you'll place fifth or sixth—on a good day! The same can be said for the outcome of your day when you're starting it in such a hopeless place.

I need you to go for the gold! Wake up in the morning and plan—even if you don't believe it—to do all the things that you know are in the best interest of your relationship. Make your food plan for the day, prep your meals, or think about where and what you'll order. Talk through what time you plan to have your three meals and a snack. Think about who you're going to connect with and which skills you'll use if the day gets tough. Even if it isn't going to be absolute perfection, setting yourself up for that scenario makes you more likely to fulfill your goals. "Shoot for the moon. Even if you miss, you'll land among the stars."

It's 4:00, and then it's 4:01

There will be some days when everything goes as planned, and, frankly, I hope that happens more often than not. Inevitably, there are days when life has other plans. That's the part of your relationship that no one talks about. Slips happen in all different shapes and sizes: Your flight is delayed and there's nowhere to eat a proper lunch; you're having friends over, so you feel "obligated" to have a bite of the cheesecake; you're working late and forget to plan dinner, so you get home and graze or snack throughout the evening; you're overwhelmed and eat five pieces of Ezekiel bread at dinner instead of the two the plan suggests; your son is eating an ice cream cone and you take a few bites without even thinking. I could go on forever.

Your reaction to the slip can no longer be torching your car and saying "game over"—or, rather, "*Game on*—I'm eating *all* the food!" That's not a sustainable solution.

It's not a question of *if* you're going to go off track—because you definitely will. Slips are going to happen; it's a simple fact of the long-term-relationship game. And in such times, you need to make a pledge: Stop slashing your tires, lighting your car on fire, and going back to square one. No more. You have choices now. The truth is that you can be doing one thing at four in the afternoon and you can be doing something completely different at 4:01. It's never too late to get back on plan, despite what the voice of your distorted perfectionism may tell you.

This is going to take resolve. It may feel like you're pulling your mind back from the gates of hell, constantly reminding yourself that you no longer need to go there. In the early days, I was told by the people supporting me in my new relationship that I was addicted to starting over—I looooved me a day one, a good restart, not realizing how toxic that was to my relationship to food—and myself! So this concept of getting right back on the minute I realize I'm off is one I've had to remind myself of over and over. I need to remember that my relationship problems weren't created out of one instance of overeating at a steak dinner, taking a few handfuls of potato chips, or adding an extra snack. They were largely born out of my *reaction* to those slips—torching the car and leaving it on the highway, instead of changing the flat and getting on with the business of my awesome life.

Shorthand for your slips: When you slip, make a corrective action plan for how to prevent it from happening again. Forgive, but certainly don't forget. That's how you keep the frequency, intensity, and duration of your slipping at a minimum. Then, get right back on plan and move on with your wonderful life, more unscathed than ever.

Byeeeeee, cheat days!

With this plan, I need you to acknowledge that slips happen, but you never, ever *intend* for them to. *Wait. What? No cheat days?!* You read that right. While amazing in theory, cheat days are a slippery slope and an awful product of your diet trauma. They lead you right back into the arms of Sugar—give the white stuff an inch and it will take a mile. Very rarely do planned cheat days last a day, and if they do, the damage done is enough for a week. Plus, living your big, exciting life will always throw you enough real-time curveballs, so making a plan to cheat—and boy do I *hate* that word, especially when we're talking about creating a loving relationship!—adds too much to the slip category.

Endgame

The entire objective of the Anti-Perfection Plan is to put you back into the best version of your relationship, as soon as possible, with minimal harm and minimal reaction. No outrageous overeating in the name of *I've already messed up.* No skipping or skimping on your next meal because you ate too much. Set your frustration, shame, and disappointment aside. Life goes on as planned.

SOMETHING IS *ALWAYS* BETTER THAN NOTHING

After reading your Relationship Rebuild Plan, you may have thought to yourself, *There's no effing way. That's not enough food for me.* Maybe that feeling made you want to rip this book to shreds, give up completely, or eat everything in sight. *I get it.* That's a totally reasonable reaction when the solution you are being offered feels impossible. It's one I've had to food plans like this for as long as I can remember. If that's what you're experiencing, please know that I feel your pain and it isn't my intent for you to feel this way. Big-time apologies.

And here's the thing: You may very well be right. The RRP is a generalized plan that was created for the average reader. The truth may be that you are not in the average category right now. Your suffering in this relationship may be more to the tune of many thousands of calories—deep and dark bottoms that makes the RRP feel like a joke to you. I understand. At my clinic, we make very individualized plans for people, depending on where they are in the recovery process. But because we don't get to be with each other in real life, I need you to make these decisions—with my full guidance and support—on your own.

Instead of focusing on what you can't do, let's focus on what you *can* do—something is *always* better than nothing. And something so often leads to bigger and better things, or in this case, greater and more positive change.

One of my most successful clients, Jason, came to the Beacon eating more than a dozen eggs for breakfast with a loaf of bread, up to forty dollars' worth of fast food for lunch, two to three pizzas at dinner . . . you get the idea. If I had suggested that he eat two eggs with a slice of cheese and a piece of toast for breakfast, I think he would have laughed in my face and fired me on the spot. I knew that Sugar and Flour needed to come out of his diet ASAP, and I knew we needed to stabilize him in a more thoughtful way than simply asking him to go from eating ten thousand calories to eighteen hundred. That was *not* a realistic or sustainable solution.

The portions could wait. Why? The Sugar and Flour were his immediate problem—the issue causing him the most harm, altering his brain and endocrine system. The *amount* of food he ate was a lower priority. And frankly, eliminating Sugar and Flour decreased his caloric intake from ten thousand to six thousand and he released a whole bunch of weight, which was of high importance to him. In time, he felt more prepared to decrease his portions, little by little. And now he's on the regular old RRP, releasing weight like a boss.

The best things come to those who wait—and all the best things can't always happen all at once. If decreasing your intake so rigorously feels too unrealistic and overwhelming, start by just removing Sugar and Flour. This will have the most dramatic impact on your recovery and will help open the gates of willingness for you to adopt more of the suggestions in the RRP. As a bonus, I've found that taking Sugar and Flour out of your diet often results in eating less anyway, even if you're not trying. So don't sweat it. Continue to work toward the guidelines outlined in chapter seven—and be cool, loving, and gentle if you feel the need to be the tortoise instead of the hare.

When you just don't wanna

Then there are times we make mistakes that are not so accidental. Let's get really real: There may be times when you don't want to follow your food plan, and you don't want to use your fancy toolbox to help you tolerate the uncomfortable feeling you're having or the situation you're in. It's too aggravating to go out of your way looking for Sugar- and Flour-free options. You get frustrated that other people don't have to do this, while you do. Or you're experiencing really big emotions that you just want to numb. There will be days when following the food plan seems impossible for many reasons. You may even feel that way right now.

As much as I hate it, there are times when *no* is the only answer available. There may be times when I could be sitting in your kitchen ready to talk things out, but your determination to binge would be so great that you'd push me out of the way. I get it.

We're going to do things differently this time. So with any little sliver of willingness you can muster up in times like these, I need you to ask yourself, "Is there anything I am willing to do in this moment that can make my binge less harmful?" Because the most important thing in this moment is to not lean into Sugar and Flour. Turn to food you love but you don't looooooooooove, if you know what I mean. Of course your impulse will be to dive into the ice cream, but can you consider starting with vegetables and hummus instead? If you're going to take a misstep, can you make them in quantity (too many veggies and hummus) rather than quality (ice cream)? Turning to Sugar or Flour in these times changes the game from emotional to chemical. This awakens your nervous and endocrine systems and puts you at greater risk to succumb to your physical addiction.

And you may fight the good fight and try with all your might in these moments, but Sugar still lures you back. Here I need you to remember that everything is reparable. Head right back to your Anti-Perfection Plan ASAP. *Code red*. If you fall in the hole, get out as soon as you can.

TAKE WHAT YOU WANT AND LEAVE THE REST

One size doesn't fit all—not in food and not in life. It's true that each person is unique, with different histories, vulnerabilities, and strengths. Like I said before, this program has worked for thousands of people who had never before found sustainable success. I'm hoping the same can be said for you.

But let's remember what we learned with the Anti-Perfection Plan: You don't have to completely abandon the plan if you're feeling that certain parts don't perfectly resonate with you. The endgame is sustainability and freedom, and the path there is going to look different for every person who breaks up with Sugar.

As the saying goes, take what you want and leave the rest. Just remember, Sugar can be sneaky and seductive. It can convince you of things that are not in your best interest. Be sure to always be considerate of your motive and your Guiding Values—be sure that what you're choosing to amend or adjust is helping you move toward your ultimate goal of a peaceful and loving relationship with food and yourself.

THE ULTIMATE GOAL: DO NO HARM

The hope and excitement that my clients experience when they learn the art of living in the gray area is nothing short of miraculous. These are *truly* the concepts that will keep you in this relationship for good, that will allow you to stay the course and not cut and run to the next diet that will inevitably fail you. And you must know and remember, *these tools are for emergency use only*.

Your abusive relationship with Sugar is rooted so deep in denial, and abuse of these skills can trigger the very same delusions. Undoubtedly, eating a bag of chips is better than eating a dozen doughnuts, but it's best that you eat neither. Eating one bite of cake is better than the whole slice, but it's best that you have none at all. *The ultimate goal of reducing harm is to do no harm.* When you're using these emergency tools, be sure to get back to your plan ASAP. This has been a public service announcement, one that I hope you will take very seriously.

I Broke Up with Sugar

Simone

I didn't have weight problems as a kid. I mean, I was always what people called "big-boned" but never really overweight. I was curvier than most of my peers and definitely a little awkward, but fat? Not really, despite how I might have felt on the inside. I always wanted to be thinner, constantly comparing myself to my sister and father, who were able to restrict themselves to seven hundred calories a day. But somehow, I could never manage to have just an apple for lunch and a salad for dinner. After all, I played tennis and swam competitively—a superactive tomboy.

I grew up in a home where addictions, secret-keeping, and silent suffering were the norm. So when my weight started to roller-coaster following a series of abandonments, I did what my family had taught us to do with feelings—I hid them, told no one, and turned right to Sugar.

It was the start of a fascination with how many gallons of ice cream—topped with Magic Shell, of course—I could eat standing over the kitchen sink in one day. And then it grew to eating whole birthday cakes and discarding the container in the neighbor's trash can so no one would be the wiser. It started to escalate as abusive relationships do: minimizing what I ate at dinner with friends so I could go home and eat the fridge in private; restricting myself all day so I could . . . eat the fridge the way I wanted to in the quantities that soothed me.

After years of bingeing and restricting, I found Molly. I learned that I didn't need to hide what I was doing anymore and could live out in the open in a community of people who share my story. I was in shock to find out that sharing my truth was healing!

While it was tough, I learned to tolerate Sugar cravings and the urges to go in on a good self-soothing binge just because I couldn't stand the thought of being uncomfortable for even a second. Removing that maniac Sugar from my life changed everything. My cravings are virtually gone—I sit next to my nephew and watch him eat ice cream without wanting even a bite. *That* is true freedom.

And I wouldn't have it without Molly and my breakup with Sugar. Don't get me wrong—this doesn't mean that I do it perfectly. Perfect doesn't exist. It can't. Not in my world. My obsession with doing everything *just so* led to *big* slips, in and out of diets that didn't work—couldn't work—because they demanded nothing but absolute perfection. The greatest knowledge came from learning how to get right back into my life and onto my plan after slips, without wanting to tear myself down, beat myself up, and essentially throw away everything I had worked for. So I stand in my truth—no Sugar, no Flour, and I've divorced dieting. And my slips are just that: slips. They are no longer slides. The truth is, the freedom that I have found in this program *and* in the imperfection of it is something I would never jeopardize again. Not ever.

I Broke Up with Sugar

Jane

I don't think I can remember a time in my life when I wasn't on a diet. I had tried no carbs on Tuesdays, no fruit on Wednesdays, counting points, food delivery, fiber crackers, and countless other attempts to lose weight and live my best life. Yet I still felt hopeless, miserable, and out of control. I was truly at the end of my rope. I felt completely unhealthy. When I heard about the program from a friend who was doing it, I was curious and intrigued, but also skeptical. *How could she be losing weight eating a potato with her dinner?* My friend encouraged me to call and set up an appointment with Molly and I said, "No, it's not for me. I like my fiber crackers." Her response was, "Great, how is that working for you?" (Well, that was eye-opening!)

When I met Molly, it was as if she knew me without knowing me. No one had ever truly understood what I was going through, because I'd honestly never told anyone. It made me too uncomfortable to talk about it, but Molly knew in the first five minutes of my twenty-minute consultation with her.

The rest is history. For the next three weeks, I plowed through and started to gain control of my life. But it wasn't until probably week four that I started to own my abusive relationship with Sugar. Not only did I learn that it is common, but I learned about why those of us who struggle with Sugar are addicted to it. I learned strategies for how to cope with potential and actual slips. In my issues with food, there is no question that can't be answered and no problem that can't be solved! That knowledge gives me tremendous comfort—this will be a lifelong endeavor. I will always be grateful to Molly for this new life, as well as my friend for not taking no for an answer.

Chapter 14

Divorcing Dieting

Ahh, happily ever after. That has a nice ring to it, doesn't it? And we are well on our way! Not to burst your bubble, but there is one more sincere separation in order. That's right—check your prenup, call the lawyers, and get ready to sign on the dotted line, because I'm going to ask you to *divorce dieting*.

Another breakup? Yes, I know. But in your heart of hearts you know it's necessary. The only other relationship that is as bad as—maybe even worse than—your relationship with Sugar and Flour is your relationship with dieting. You know all too well the deceptive lure of a new diet: the rapid results, the quick fix, the one-and-done. I can feel that enticing rush just writing about it! New, shiny packaging and irresistible promises! It's all so sexy and appealing, making it almost impossible not to fall into the trap. Like any fun fling, joyride, hot romp in the hay, diets offer us simple and easy promises—promises that they can't actually keep.

Way back in the first chapter of this book, I asked you to consider taking the Sacred Vow, on which the bedrock of your new relationship with food and with yourself would be built. I asked you to consider staying the course—to let go of your awful and destructive habit of cutting and running when things get hard, to give up your "chronic cheater" status that you've earned along this rocky relationship path. Remember that?

Divorcing dieting is saying you are done dating the proverbial "bad boys." You know the type. The relationship that's thrilling at first glance but in actuality is just infuriating and tormenting. You can always count on being swept off your feet with grandiose promises—"This time, it will be different." But it never is. It's always followed by a roller coaster of emotions, disappointments, crying jags, powwows with your friends. But it always ends with a big flaming breakup, leaving you war-torn and hopeless.

Exhausting, isn't it? That's the cycle of dieting and it's as destructive as your relationship with Sugar. Your wisest self knows that the "bad boys" are not healthy for you and don't help you get any closer to your relationship goals. Yet you go back. And back. And back again.

You may be thinking, *Molly, I'm convinced. I've hit my rock bottom. I'm staying broken up with Sugar and Flour. We're good to go.* And while I'm beyond excited that you're trending toward living and loving in your new relationship, the seductive lure of dieting is stronger than you can ever imagine. Just wait until your friend loses weight on an easy-and-fast diet and tells you just how simple it is, or you get disappointed that you're not releasing weight fast enough, or you have a particularly hard day filled with hating your food plan and hating how you look, or you slip and decide that this breakup just isn't working. Remember, these feelings are temporary (and, sadly, so is your friend's success on her diet du jour). I know I sound like a broken record, but *they will pass.* You need to know the truth about dieting so that you can stay divorced, turn to your plan and skills, and not be lured to cut and run from your beautiful relationship.

WHY DO I DO THIS?

As humans, we have very vulnerable brains. The diet industry knows this all too well. I could write a separate book about the time and money it spends figuring out what to say to you in the name of selling you another fad. We live in a world of "diet porn"—what's being sold to you is bigger, faster, and more extreme than what the actual solution could ever hope to offer. When you're desperate for a solution, of course you're going to gravitate toward lofty and enticing promises: "Fifteen pounds in fifteen days!" "Drink this tea for an instant flat belly!" "Lose the weight and eat all the foods you love!" These magic "solutions" are unrealistic, highly improbable, and certainly not sustainable. You've become so accustomed to seeing these messages, your expectations have gotten completely out of whack. Reminder: Bigger, faster, and more extreme is *not* always better.

My diet drama and trauma days were an absolute mess. You know the story all too well: Ninety-nine times out of one hundred I would lose my grip on the diet du jour with an epic binge, gaining back any weight I had lost plus a bunch of extra pounds. But that's not the story I need to shed light on. The story we need to focus on is my—and your—reaction to that *one time out of one hundred* when I seemingly had success. Because *that's* what keeps us hooked and going back for more.

You know those "shooting-star moments"—by some grace you're able to hold on for dear life and follow the plan, lose a bunch of weight, and manage to keep it off for a month, maybe even a year. Because failure and disappointment are the normal feelings you experience with dieting, these "successes" stand out in your mind and tower above everything else—including those other ninety-nine times you failed miserably. With this glimpse of "success" at the forefront of your consciousness, you are drawn back into the diet craze, despite the unfavorable odds. Would you get into a car that had crashed every time you took it out except once? What about if it crashed 50 percent of the time? You still wouldn't do it. By continuing to diet, you're banking your new relationship on something that's likely to crash and burn, leaving your hormones, metabolism, and self-esteem wrecked and mangled beyond recognition. Pretty crazy, right? *There was that one time ten years ago when I lost thirty pounds on that conventional diet program. I know I gained forty-five back, but if I could just do that one more time. . . .*

In this way, diets are *exactly* like abusive relationships. And that one out of a hundred is hazardous—to your relationship and to your life. You know that first big weigh-in when we tell ourselves, "This is *exactly* what my relationship with food and weight should be"? I'm always amazed how, with that one number drop, we forget all the disappointment, suffering, and demoralization that past diets have caused us and celebrate the idea that we're not a hopeless case.

Here's where you need to understand *intermittent reinforcement*. It's a term used in psychology to explain what happens when rewards are given inconsistently. And that's what has you hooked—hard-core—into your relationship with dieting.

Intermittent reinforcement is used with slot machines and video games to keep people plugging away—you pour your money into the machines, waiting for the jackpot, believing that the next pull will be the big winner and all your problems will be fixed. Your relationship is even more complicated if you've hit a jackpot before or have a friend who has won the lotto: *I know I can do it again. I just need one more shot.*

Abusive relationships function the very same way. Even though your partner screams at you and calls you names, there are selective times when they buy you flowers and shower you with loving compliments. You stay in the relationship despite the damage, waiting for the few occasions you feel cared for and appreciated. "But you don't understand," you say. "They can be so sweet and loving." The same can be said for your dieting dependency. Despite periods of despair, frustration, and failure, you stick around for that rare moment when you experience some weight loss. All the while, you're unwittingly getting pulled deeper and deeper into the fantasy of the dieting ideal.

THE DARK SIDE OF DIETING

Have you ever started a diet and found yourself unintentionally lured into bingeing on low-fat, low-cal chocolate chip muffins or an all-natural acai bowl? So many "diet foods" turn out to be extraordinarily triggering and actually lock you into your problematic relationship with food. They promote the idea that you can have it all ("Eat all the foods you know and love, and still lose weight!") But they are actually just helping to keep you hooked on Flour and Sugar.

Worst of all, dieting cements you to your bingeing and compulsive overeating. You know how we love a good reward? Science tells us that not only do we like rewards, we are actually hyperresponsive to them; it feels like they completely take over our brain space. Periods of heavy restriction—which is virtually every diet you've ever done—make us more vulnerable to cravings and urges to overeat. When we finally give in, torching the particular diet we've pledged to, our brain is anxiously waiting for its reward.

Our brains *expect* a reward every time we cut and run from one diet to the next! Bouncing from restrictive diet to restrictive diet, depriving yourself of calories and nutrients and putting added stress on your body, unintentionally primes your brain for binge eating. Who knew dieting had this dark of a dark side?

Oh, the FOMO!

So many things feel scary when we're talking about ditching dieting. Even though you know you're doing what's absolutely best for you, you're also deciding to not participate in one of the biggest cultural norms. And that will cue *all* the FOMO: Fear of Missing Out.

FOMO was coined by Harvard MBA Patrick J. McGinnis. He describes it as "the desire to stay constantly connected to the actions of others and the latest trends." What puts gasoline on the flame of FOMO? Social media and online marketing.

You know it's true: Every time you scroll through your feed, you are constantly inundated with marketing ploys to get you hooked on the latest trend. It should come as no surprise that social media has contributed to the diet industry earning sixty-six billion dollars a year on the back of your FOMO. Detoxes and weight-loss products are taking over Instagram, while Cardi B and the Kardashians are being paid to tell you how your life will change with a lollipop or cup of tea. Other products claim to detox your body without any science to back it up. Deep down you know something's up—these products *must* contain something like stimulants, laxatives, or diuretics, which all come with some hefty detrimental consequences from long-term use. But with the glittering promise of a flat stomach and glamorous life, *despite knowing the real truth*, you're back in the game—I WANT *THAT*.

I WANT THAT *NOW*. Add impatience to the perfect storm of FOMO and the internet, and you have a real situation on your hands— one that will derail your long-term relationship goals fast. Getting sucked into the whirlpool of our fast-paced world will tickle every part of you that wants the quick fix right now. It will convince you that the sustainable solution you've been nurturing is too hard, too tedious, too boring, too long-term, too slow, too everything . . . The seduction of a thirty-day detox or a fourteen-pounds-in-fourteen-days plan will trigger every part of your commitment issues. It will incite you to get your matches and set this amazing, loving relationship on fire. So be prepared with your wisdom, your commitment . . . and your fire extinguisher.

Beware of the seduction

Even if everything you've read in this book makes good, logical sense, there are a lot of triggers that can pull you back to diets. You've become accustomed to acting like a chronic cheater in your relationship with food, and old habits are hard to break. This relationship you're building with food is still very new, so it's understandable you may be quite vulnerable to the seduction of dieting. It's to be expected, and we need to prepare you.

Think of what it will be like to silently watch your friends and colleagues on the next big sexy diet, while you're chilling on your RRP, business as usual. Maybe your friend shares a weight-loss story: "You will never believe how much weight this girl lost on this diet. Must have been like fifty pounds in three months! She made it seem so easy. I could hardly believe it!" You then think, *Wow, that could be me. Maybe I should ditch my RRP and do what this girl is doing. If it worked for her, it must work for me!* Giving up dieting can make you feel like a real outsider, and it can also be frustrating at times when it *seems* like others are getting results faster and more easily than you.

Speaking of "faster," how annoying is it when the scale doesn't move as fast as you want it to? The disappointment, frustration, and sadness that you may feel when you're not releasing weight as quickly as your previous "starvation diets" may seduce you into ditching the long game for the short-term satisfaction of quick fixes. When we feel frustrated, we're compelled to respond with drastic action. *This is what got you into this situation to begin with.*

The last thing I want to prepare you for are the emotions that will inevitably come if you slip. After your first misstep, you may think, *See? This program isn't working. I would be better off sticking to a strict diet.* It would be *utterly ridiculous* to expect you to be perfect in your new life; it makes absolutely no sense to burn the whole house down if you've only clogged the toilet.

Love and peace, your new normal

Even with all this intel on demonic dieting, I'd guess you're still feeling pretty hooked in. Just like you've grieved the loss of Sugar, you will most certainly grieve this loss. Diets have helped you believe there is a quick fix to your problems.

So many of my clients balk at the maintenance phase of their breakup with Sugar. *What's the endgame?* They're frightened of the potential monotony of this life—how dull and unexciting life feels without the high of finding an easier, quicker fix, the instability of yo-yo dieting. They fear the B word, *boredom.*

And I guess this peaceful, loving, guilt- and worry-free life could be categorized as boring—at least right now, given you've spent the majority of your life chronically dieting and seeking the next savior/abuser. All that instability has molded you into a chaos junkie! It will definitely feel a little empty having less noise and chaos surrounding your food, body, and weight—that will take some getting used to. But your trade-off will be the peace and love you'll become accustomed to and the everyday moments in which you'll find joy.

One of my dearest friends, Julie, dated bad boy after bad boy for decades. One day, she met Matt, who is one of the nicest, kindest, most available and giving men I know. When she decided to take the plunge and go all in with him, Julie said, "I had to accept that I was never going to get into a knockdown-drag-out fight with amazing, intense makeup sex. This loving calm was going to be my new normal." It took her a minute to adjust to this new life of hers, and it will probably take you a minute to adjust, too. Of course it will—you've practiced this toxic dance of dieting, detoxing, more dieting, and cleansing for your whole life! Gone will be the thrill of starting a new diet on January 1, juice cleansing before a big event, or joining your company's thirty-day weight-loss challenge. Like my friend Julie, you're going to have to get used to this new normal.

Now it's time to decide if you can pledge to yourself—take the leap; make the solemn promise to yourself and the relationships you are creating to *divorce dieting*. Breaking up with Sugar and Flour heals and rebuilds your relationship with food. Divorcing dieting—staying the course of this new relationship you are creating no matter what—is what heals your relationship with *yourself*.

I Broke Up with Sugar

Christine

My love affair with Sugar began at the tender age of five. Every Sunday, we would spend time at my grandmother's house. She had a closet in the kitchen full of candy, which included a tin canister full of M&M's. That's how M&M's became my go-to for whatever I was feeling that day, whether sad, happy, lonely, confused, or just plain hungry.

Over the years, my love affair with Sugar in the form of candy, cookies, cake, and pie continued to grow. But I was never heavy; despite my abusive relationship with Sugar, I was always able to maintain a normal weight. That is, until my late thirties. That's when the trouble began. Doing graduate school, raising young children, and working, I gained a hundred pounds. Whatever I was feeling that day, I believed Sugar would make it better. I was feeling terrible about myself and made what seemed like a million attempts to lose weight. I joined Weight Watchers more times than I can count. I would lose some weight and then gain it all back. I loved to get weighed on Saturday so I could eat all weekend and then try to lose whatever I gained and then some more before my next weigh-in. It was a perpetual cycle of eating, trying to lose, eating more, and trying to lose again, and it was never successful.

Then I met Molly. Believe me when I tell you breaking up with Sugar was not easy, but it is the best thing I have ever done for myself and my family. Molly gave me the tools to understand why Sugar was not my friend. Understanding the science behind what Sugar does to me is what I needed. I grieved like I'd just lost my best friend, and I was pissed about the fact that I was and will always be addicted to my beloved Sugar. I raged, I screamed, I asked, "Why me?" a million times. I went through withdrawal and came out on the other side.

Today, I feel better than I have ever felt in my life. Everything has changed. I've also divorced dieting—no more starting a diet on January 1 or the Tuesday after Labor Day or any given Monday. I don't think about food constantly like I used to and am much more focused in my job. I have healthier relationships with my family and feel so much better about myself. I owe so much to Molly for helping me make my life what it is today. I will always be grateful.

Chapter 15

Finding Freedom in Humble Eating

There are two relationships you cannot avoid in life: the one you have with food and the one you have with yourself. I'll never stop reminding you of this. These are relationships you cannot escape, and ideally you shouldn't want to! In their finest form, they will bring you joy, peace, and comfort and they will be the bedrock of your beautiful life.

In that spirit, we need to discuss the question I'm asked over and over again: "So, this breakup with Sugar and Flour—it's for the rest of my life? I have to follow this plan forever?" My first answer to this question is: "Forever is a really long time." And my second is: "Yes . . . sort of."

If you're fully engaged in your RRP, living by your vows and your Guiding Values, and using skills like a boss, then you're probably feeling pretty good these days. Maybe you're even moving toward (gasp!) acceptance that this can be a far better life than you could have imagined. Not going to say I told you so . . .

RENT TO OWN

But here's the thing: I've given you the model that's worked amazingly for so many people. In that way, you're in the "renting" stage of your new life—being compliant, following the guidelines and vows that were prescribed for you. And I love you for that. You can't even begin to know how awesome you are. I love that you've taken your vow to have an open mind so seriously in creating this new relationship. And I know it's going to pay really high dividends.

Now it's time to move from compliance to acceptance. From renting to owning. Your new relationship with food needs to have *your* stamp of approval, which will transition the full ownership to you. It's what turns this process from a short-term diet to a long-term relationship. With your newfound experience and wisdom in determining what works for you, a deeper and more profound understanding of your relationship with food and, just as important, with yourself will develop.

Our pal research is in complete agreement when it comes to this process of ownership, or as we call it in my business, *self-determination*. In fact, with all the conflicting information floating around in the world of food and weight, the research on self-determination is one piece of data that is pretty unflappable.

The headline of self-determination theory says that for you to thrive and prosper in this new life you're creating, the motivation needs to come from *within you*, because when a change is rigid and prescribed, you're far less likely to stick to it. When you have a more active and independent choice and your motivation is deep-seated, you're more likely to change for good. Research also tells us that those with self-determination have better outcomes, including successful eating regulation, increased physical activity, greater weight loss after treatment, and long-term maintenance. That's why you need to add that special blend of *you* to really own this new relationship.

WHAT IS HUMBLE EATING?

Practicing humility means knowing your strengths, understanding your limitations, and acting accordingly. The importance of humility in this process of ownership is what led me to call this concept *humble eating*. It's my greatest wish that on this journey, should you want to, you can loosen the reins and humbly practice flexibility in your new relationship with food.

Obviously, I'm not suggesting that humble eating means cake and pizza for breakfast. And let me be clear that there is a ginormous difference between giving yourself permission to slip (which is most definitely not something you want to get into the habit of) and accessing your inner wisdom. Be mindful of impulsivity trying to pretend that it's good judgment.

Humble eating is not picking off your kid's plate because you haven't had dinner yet, or taking a bite of food you know will trigger you to want more. That's why having some bottom-line behaviors and guidelines—ones you know work for you, that help to keep you rocking your best self and give some needed structure to your life—is paramount to this relationship. As is being willing to turn back to the fundamentals of the plan if you've given yourself too much rope. That's what they're there for, and that's the humble choice.

After sixty-six days of living your vows and following your RRP, your mind will be far more clear than when we first started this journey. This may be a great time to investigate what's working for you and what isn't. What's feeling too restrictive and what's feeling really warm and nurturing. What's bringing you closer to the relationship of your dreams and what's making you pine for the days of yore when Sugar and Flour were by your side.

Maybe in your breakup with Sugar and Flour you found it difficult to go out to dinner because the environment presented too many potential triggers, but after sixty-six days, you want to try to live more freely and dine out with more frequency. Or maybe the breakup with Sugar and Flour was easy for you, but the volume has been a sticking point, so you want to continue to focus on your portions. Maybe eating four times a day isn't working for you and you think eating three or five times a day suits you best. Maybe you'll find that your relationship with Sugar was so abusive that fruit is something you feel triggered by and choose not to eat, or that your relationship with Flour isn't so bad and you feel like you can try chickpea pasta or almond flour. Maybe you have no issue with alcohol and can be more flexible with the suggested two-drink maximum. Maybe your problems with missing Sugar only come when the clock strikes eight, and that's where you need to draw a hard line on ending your day's eating. The list is truly endless.

Here's the thing. You may remove your snack to find that you're more obsessed with food, or try chickpea pasta and feel hungrier than ever, or find that you are gaining weight with all that dining out. Guess what? Your foundational plan—your vows and your RRP—are always waiting for you if you get off track. Your answer will always be the same: Head back to your true north for a while. Once you return to basics and feel like you're on solid ground again, you can make the decision—if you are feeling the pull—to try something else that feels right to you.

Adding humble eating to your relationship . . . humbly

Now for the question of *when* to add humble eating to your relationship. It's an advanced skill, without a doubt; it may take some time before you're ready to fly without the map I've created for you. As much as I'd love to promise you a magic number of when that day will come, I know that in good conscience I can't. Everyone is walking different paths, with unique circumstances that make each journey distinct.

What I can tell you with certainty is that once you've put in the legwork of serious repetition with your new food and food behaviors, some wonderful things will start to happen. Remember back in previous chapters when I shared the research about habits forming at the sixty-six-day mark? We're going to use that as a benchmark. If you've committed to breaking up with Sugar, following a meal plan, and weighing and measuring your food to the best of your ability, then you can expect your food foundation to solidify in about sixty-six days. But that, my friend, is a *minimum*.

One size does not fit all, and one number does not address the complexities of your brain, the severity of your abusive relationship with Sugar and Flour, your diet drama and trauma—the list of individual sensitivities is endless. This path to creating a loving relationship with food will look a little different for everyone. Some of you may take sixty-six days on the mark, some ninety, some a year. I've known people who took up to five years to solidify these habits (but that was after *many* stops and starts, allowing Sugar back in *just this once*). But even they did it. And it worked.

Healing a relationship like this is a lot like healing a bone. Your doctor will immobilize it for six weeks and put you in a cast. I hope at the six-week mark you wouldn't just go rip off your cast and run a marathon! You'd head back to the doctor, get an assessment, and follow the recommendations you were given. And, as is sometimes the case, you might be told that your bone needs more time to recover.

We all heal differently. And we all heal at our own pace. When you find yourself firmly planted in your food foundation and it feels like you're in a really solid rhythm, then you may be ready to transition into humble eating.

If you never leave basics, you never have to go back to basics

Side note: Humble eating isn't for everyone. Plenty of people, at least over the short run, do best renting and *not* owning. They do best following someone else's instructions and not complicating their new relationship with experiments. After years and years of diet roller-coaster drama and trauma, you may be the happiest little clam with your RRP, your vows, and your skills. If that's the case, good for you! If you never leave basics, you never need to go back to basics, so stay there as long as you'd like! It's pretty advanced to know that the basics work for you and that you're not interested in making things more complicated.

Making sure humble eating doesn't turn on you

You're giving yourself some rope to explore your relationship. Let's just make sure you're not taking so much that you hang yourself. There's a fine line between humble eating and full-blown relapse. Your relationship with Sugar is rooted deeply in delusion: *It's fine. It's no big deal. I'm humble eating! I'll just have a little.*

Humble eating requires being awake and aware. You don't get to *not* pay attention. If you are not mindful in this relationship, it *will* turn on you. We want this relationship to be loving and freeing, not reinjuring. For that to happen, keep your humility intact, pay attention to any red flags, and don't ignore the foundation you've worked so hard to build.

The humility in humble eating is the knowledge that your bliss lies in always maintaining some structure in your relationship. What that looks like will be different for everyone, and it will certainly change and grow as you change and grow. It will mean always having your eye on your relationship with Sugar and Flour—knowing the foods and food behaviors that work and those that inflict harm. It's checking in with yourself asking, "Is this food taking me out of my life or is it helping me to be in my life?" If you've eaten more than you've intended, feel physically or emotionally unwell postgame, or think about when and where you can next get more, the food is likely ruling the roost again. In order for humble eating to help you thrive and grow, you need to be willing to take a closer look at your behaviors to make sure you're on the path to success, not on the road back to your abusive relationship with Sugar.

FEAR OF FOREVER

Do I have to do this forever? This is the most common of the fears that people struggle with on this journey. I don't know what anyone should do forever, but I do know that if you have identified with anything I've written in this book, you need to stay humbly aware that you'll always require some sort of framing around your food. That's the price of entry into this big beautiful life you're approaching.

My clients who practice humble eating have a general idea of their meal plan for each day. They all have different versions of the plan—some have added a snack, some have removed the snack, some have four drinks in a week, some have added more fat into their plan (okay, that's me), some more protein, and some allow themselves a handful of potato chips from time to time since their weight was released. Some never measure their food, some only measure their nuts (okay, that one is me, too). All of them look back to their 66-day vows and their plan when their pants get a little tighter, when they are short with their spouses, or when they are just feeling generally "off." And sometimes they camp out there for a week or a month or a year. All the humble eaters know what works, they know what doesn't, and they act accordingly. And they know that what *doesn't* work is hoovering containers of cookie dough. And should some cookie dough find its way into their stomachs, they know to get back to their plan ASAP.

In living a big, fun, adventurous life, I find myself in situations that are tricky beyond measure. Don't cry for me—they're usually in beautiful locales where there's not a lot of individual choice when it comes to food. There are situations where I don't get to decide mealtimes, and when there are meals, they are gorgeous but filled with heavy, high-calorie food. Of course, I do my best—I never slash tires. I'm always thinking, always trying to stay true to my plan despite the circumstances. And yet, my portions are usually larger and I am eating foods, albeit Sugar- and Flour-free, that I don't eat on the regular. And as much fun as I have on these trips—and I have *fun!*—the minute I set foot in my home, I'm back on my RRP and back in the vows. I find them to be nurturing, relaxing, and comforting, not punishing or confining. It's how I practice humble eating and get all the things I want out of life.

The best news of all is that humble eating helps you keep your focus on food when it's time to eat, and on your life when the eating is done. Leading with humility is a very empowered way to live.

So when you ask, "Do I have to do this forever—for the rest of my life?" I hope my answer, "Yes . . . sort of," makes more sense. You have to be in a relationship with food forever—that's where the *yes* comes in. But it can be one in which you create a flexible structure, with some supports to protect you when times get tough. Humble eating is about finding more peace and freedom, allowing for your relationships with yourself and with food to grow and thrive in the way that best suits *you*.

Right now is the best place to live

All this talk about humble eating and experimenting with more or less or different can light your sense of wonder and adventure on fire. It can tap right into your compulsive dieting and desire to cut and run to something "better." I have to share humble eating with you now, because I don't know if we'll still be besties in two months and six days' time, and I want to impart all the knowledge while I have you.

It's super important that we focus *all* of our attention on the most effective place to live, which is in the here and now. And in the here and now, I want to give you a sweet and loving reminder that humble eating is for *after* you've mastered the fundamentals of your RRP and the skills. It's a way of life you may choose *after* your sixty-six days of healing, refocusing, and resetting. So, right now, please try to give your mind a break from thinking about this next step and let the sixty-six days do its thing. Then you can humbly decide your next steps.

I Broke Up with Sugar

Therese-Ann

I've started and stopped diets for years. You could even say I'm a diet expert. I knew the points of every food item that ever entered my mouth, I'd order my salad dressing on the side and modestly dip my fork in it as opposed to pouring it on my greens. I swapped raw sugar for white, because it was "healthier." I'd choose the salmon and forgo the fries. I'd approach every Monday as a new opportunity to "be good," while adding heaps of agave to my two cups of morning coffee. Then usually by two p.m., I'd visit the candy drawer in the office for a quick hit of Swedish Fish or chocolate. The rationalizations abounded: *They're miniatures so it's okay. Agave is natural so it's healthy.* I made annual donations to the gym (paying and not going), paid my trainer for two sessions a week, and read all the books and articles on the latest and greatest fads and miracles to enter the market. All these dieting attempts led to feelings of disappointment, anger, and frustration. I felt self-loathing at my perceived inability to finish what I'd started and wondered why I lacked the discipline that would enable me to succeed. Turns out I didn't lack it; I just could not fully tap into it under a cloud of Sugar.

And then I met Molly. From the first moment, I felt like I was becoming reacquainted with a dear old friend. She totally got me. After that initial meeting, I left the office inspired, excited, maybe a little doubtful, but mostly very hopeful.

Writing here today, I have been doing the plan for over three years. I learned that for me, Sugar and Flour are my "drugs." I no longer fuss with calorie counts, I can keep my coffee and enjoy it with milk, I don't take supplements, and I don't drink hot water with lemon and cayenne pepper. While breaking up with Flour and Sugar has been hard, it's also been easier than I ever imagined it could be. It's all true—everything people write and say: that the cravings go away, that you feel *so* good, you can't even imagine putting that crap back into your body. My skin is clearer and brighter. My hair is shinier. My waistline and good curves are back. My energy is way up. My clarity of thought has significantly improved (buh-bye, Sugar fog). And the arthritis that has pained me for years post-chemo rarely bothers me at all anymore.

And it's been fun, too! I love cooking and have had a blast adapting old family recipes, experimenting with all the wonders of real, delicious food. Through this process, I have learned how to be kind to myself and my body, let go of unhelpful comparisons, stop shaming myself—even becoming my own cheerleader—and release my fixation on the scale (the scale doesn't tell you how much your heart and soul weigh). No Sugar, no Flour, and much less booze. I have never felt better.

Chapter 16

The Recipe for a Love That Lasts

You've signed up for an LTR (long-term relationship). One that lasts, the forever kind, the kind that requires a specific recipe and attention to the process of creating and maintaining your love.

Happily ever after is a real possibility when it comes to the status of your new relationship. This may very well be the best decision you'll make in your life. So let's get you set up to rejoice in all that your big beautiful life has to offer now that Sugar and Flour are out of the picture.

Together we're going to create your Relationship Recipe, which will set you up for success. We're going to plan ahead, step-by-step, for all the things that will strengthen your new relationship with food and yourself, as well as for the situations that may get in the way. We're going to talk about the things that solidify your progress in the name of sustaining your relationship. We're also going to plan for what will creep in and try to tear it down. The greatest news is that the payoff of this preparation is huge—you'll get what you put in now and way more down the line. You'll come out stronger on the other end. I'm so excited for you!

We all want to say, "Yay! I did it! No more work to do!" But let's get real: There isn't a relationship worth having in this world that is "no maintenance"—in fact, the best ones require effort and attention to thrive. Your adventure with your food and yourself is no different. So in many ways, this is the most important part of the book. I know, I know, I say that a lot, but I really mean it every time! This is the part where you learn not just how to stay broken up with Sugar and Flour but also how to thrive in your new relationship with food. This is where you learn to solidify your behaviors—making them second nature—to stay immersed in the life you're working so hard to create.

In the past, conversations and plans for living your best life with food have been limited to what you're supposed to eat and what you're not allowed to eat. Period. This time is different. We're going to plan your success and anticipate your setbacks *before they happen*, allowing you to participate in your relationship with knowledge, foresight, and clarity. There will be no need to worry about how you're going to do this, especially when it's hard, or how you're going to stay on track. You will handle all those scary unknowns in advance, because you're the designer of your new beautiful life.

The recipe for your new relationship's success requires some attention. You want to make sure you're always moving in the direction of your long-term goals, making this relationship the best it can be. You know how a mindless dash of salt can inadvertently turn into a handful, making an otherwise delicious recipe inedible. We don't want that happening here. That's why it's so important that you create your relationship recipe today and reevaluate it regularly. In your relationship's first year, I would strongly suggest you take a look at the recipe you're using *at least monthly, if not weekly* — create a ritual! Mark your calendar and set aside time to reflect on where you are, how you feel, how you want to feel, and where you want to go. See if it needs adjustments, reductions, or new ingredients. Over time, you'll find a rhythm that works for you, but I would recommend, after that first year, doing this evaluation no less than every three months—once a quarter—so you don't end up unknowingly adding or subtracting ingredients that are essential to your flourishing life. This is how we are going to build the life you deserve—by making sure you're using the elements that bring you closer to all the things you want and desire.

ROCKING YOUR RELATIONSHIP RECIPE

The best recipes balance guidelines with intuition—and this one will be no different. We want to carefully blend what works for you, what you enjoy, where your potential pitfalls lie, and where your values lie. And while no relationship will look the same as any other, the foundation on which you create your recipe will be constant, with six main areas:

- Nonnegotiables
- Orange Flags
- Power Circle
- Must-Have Skills
- Guiding Values and Personal Commitment Statement
- Joy

NONNEGOTIABLES

This is the basis of your entire relationship's success. You know your relationship with food is about your feelings, your values, and your beliefs. But if we're not talking about your food and food behaviors, we don't have anything to talk about. In order to create a recipe that will resonate with you and bring you success, incorporating what works for you and the foods that love you back is going to be absolutely essential. But we're going to take this a step further—by identifying ingredients for this recipe that are nonnegotiable. Knowing your must-have behaviors helps to take the guesswork out when times are tough; it gives you a solid and reliable base to go back to and depend on.

I compel you to channel the most open and honest part of you when making decisions about your nonnegotiables. Remember how easy it is for denial and delusion to perk up and tell you: *Everything is fine. . . . That's not so bad. . . . It's really not that big a deal. . . . You can handle it.* Those rationalizations are a large part of what got you into relationship trouble in the first place. Try your best to keep them at bay when doing this exercise. In fact, I might err on the side of safety and integrity when setting these limits. Remember, great relationships come from solid foundations. And you can always negotiate them next time you check in.

Check off the nonnegotiables that allow for your current relationship to grow and thrive. Remember, this is ever evolving—it can change in a month, three months, a year, or five years.

Your Vows

Abstaining from:

- ☐ Sugar
- ☐ Artificial sweetener
- ☐ Liquid calories (juice, smoothies, coconut water, etc.)
- ☐ Limits on alcohol and other drugs

Specify: _____

- ☐ Flour
- ☐ Mindfulness of food volume
- ☐ Weighing and measuring food

What foods? _____

- ☐ Eating every 3 to 4.5 hours
- ☐ No grazing, picking, bites, or tastes between meals
- ☐ Meal planning
- ☐ Grocery shopping

When?_____**How often?**_____

- ☐ Regular weighing:

How often?_____

Long-Lasting Skills

- ☐ Connecting with others

Specify: Who and how often?_____

- ☐ Meditation practice

How long and how often?_____

- ☐ Gratitude practice

How?_____

- ☐ Movement and breath:

How often? _____

Other Nonnegotiables

- ☐ _____
- ☐ _____
- ☐ _____
- ☐ _____
- ☐ _____
- ☐ _____

ORANGE FLAGS

Orange flags? *Don't you mean red flags, Molly?* Nope. I want you to begin to identify what your *orange* flags are, so you never have to deal with red flags again. It's way easier to adjust your behavior when things are code orange than to wait until they turn code red.

Every relationship has warning signs when things are going astray; this one is no different. A relationship doesn't go off the rails in one fell swoop. There are *always* warning signs that things aren't going as you hoped, that your relationship is taking a turn toward gloom and doom. In relationships that end poorly, these warning signs are usually ignored.

Not in this relationship! We're going to pay attention to these little behaviors as though they are big ones. I know how hard you're working to rebuild here, so let's make sure you learn from your past mistakes and beat them to the punch. The more aware you are of the thoughts, feelings, behaviors, and situations that have the power to take you off course, the more equipped you will be to resolve them.

What are the signs that will tell you that your food foundation is becoming shaky, that you may need to rework the recipe or ask for some extra help and guidance? It can be boiled down to the thoughts, feelings, behaviors, and situations that make you feel vulnerable to going back to Sugar and Flour. Take a moment to consider your last attempts at managing your food and weight. What went wrong? What took you off track? What made you prone to cutting and running back to Sugar? There are a few examples below to illustrate what this can look like:

Thoughts: *I've totally got this. I don't need to plan. One bite won't hurt. It's just a little. Ugh, I don't want to do this forever. Honey is natural; it's not really like having sugar.*

Feelings: *Overwhelmed, tired, remorseful, anxious, excited, relieved* (yup, sometimes positive feelings can lead you astray, too)

Behaviors: *"Tasting" your kid's ice cream, eating off your partner's plate, random handfuls of nuts throughout the day, waiting too long to eat and overeating, exercising as compensation (a.k.a. "working out after overeating.")*

Situations: *Going on vacation with friends, visiting your family for holidays, dinners with work colleagues, having to hang out with people who will push food on you ("Come on, just have a little cheesecake!")*

Knowing and accepting your orange flags helps your relationship thrive! Be sure to write them down and have them handy, adding to your list if any more pop up.

POWER CIRCLE

Having a Power Circle is a must, and I mean an absolute *must*. Your Power Circle is your gateway to connecting with others. In your Power Circle exist the people and communities who will support you in your relationship, serving as your encouragement, your truth tellers, your shoulders to lean on.

Your Power Circle provides you with a sense of safety, support, and connection. You might call upon your mother, cousin, daughter, friends, coach, therapist, church community, workplace, peer-support group, 12-step fellowship, book club, Zumba class, or online community. As I've said before, the list is endless, but you *must* find your tribe.

Your Power Circle also consists of the people who are rooting for you and celebrating your victories. They support you in your long-term goals and believe in your success. They are *not* the friend who says, "Come on! You mean you really won't share this pizza with me?"

No matter who is in your circle, it's important to surround yourself with people you can reach out to in a moment of crisis. If you find yourself daydreaming about picking up a chocolate croissant from your favorite bakery on the way home from work or catch yourself diving elbow-deep into the candy jar at work, it's your job to reach out to your Power Circle immediately for help.

No more silence and no more secrets. When we sit on these thoughts and feelings and stew in secrecy, we cut ourselves off from connection. And you know when Sugar likes to slither back in? When we feel disconnected and isolated. The most powerful lesson I've learned is that *none of us can do this alone.*

Make a list of the people in your Power Circle. I keep mine in my phone, just in case I don't know who to call when things start feeling tough. If you don't have a Power Circle, get on it! Take a step today to reach out to a friend who you know struggles with food, find an in-person support group, and join me on my website, mollycarmel.com, where you can stay active in this book's community.

MUST-HAVE SKILLS

In chapter nine, we walked through all the skills you can use to make hard moments tolerable, get through cravings, and better manage your emotions. Your Long-Lasting Skills (connection, meditation, movement, and breath) guide your new relationship, and they are equally as important as your Right-Now Skills (distraction, soothing, and emergency activities) to fall back on in the tough moments. You've been dating these skills for a while now, so you have some idea of which ones are most useful to you and which ones you need to hone so that you're even more skilled when the going gets rough.

In the interest of your relationship's ultimate success, I want you to have the skills you love on hand, as well as a list of the skills that need some research and practice. It's a great idea to check back in with this list and revise it as often as you can!

SKILLS I USE ALL THE TIME

Long-Lasting

1.

2.

3.

Right Now

1.

2.

3.

SKILLS I WANT TO TRY
Long-Lasting
1.
2.
3.

Right Now
1.
2.
3.

SKILLS THAT NEED MORE PRACTICE
Long-Lasting
1.
2.
3.

Right Now
1.
2.
3.

GUIDING VALUES AND PERSONAL COMMITMENT STATEMENT

This is the biggie. Your Guiding Values, which you developed in chapter twelve, will always help to steer you in the direction of your best life. They will be the driving force of your recipe's success.

You need to know what your Guiding Values are at all times. This is even more important than knowing your zip code, social security number, or last name. When you're not acting in the spirit of your Guiding Values, the feelings of shame, self-loathing, and disappointment reappear in seconds flat. It's these feelings that make you so vulnerable to the quick-fix seduction of Sugar and Flour. So when you're feeling confused in the relationship, ask yourself, "What behaviors do I need to address so I can act in accordance with my Guiding Values?" You'll be amazed at how quickly things will change when you take action.

Along with your Guiding Values, creating a personal commitment statement has proven to be something that has helped my clients stay on course and true to their integrity.

Similar to your Why, a personal commitment statement is a go-to slogan, or mantra, you can have on hand when you've lost your way. It's a helpful tool to refocus and remotivate you when your relationship is faltering. It answers the questions: What is my purpose in this relationship? Why am I doing this?

When you're not feeling aligned—when there's a sense that something is either missing or overdone, as is often the case with recipes—your Guiding Values and personal commitment statement are there to serve as a compass to guide you back to your truest self. These two course correctors will help you through hard times without you feeling the need to reopen the door to your abusive relationship with Sugar.

Make sure you have these close to you, so you can rely on and refer to them often.

JOY

Finding joy may seem like a side note, a very optional piece of this new relationship. Nothing could be further from the truth. Removing Sugar from your life leaves you with a giant void. It's especially important that you start thinking about how you're going to nourish and nurture yourself and experience joy in ways other than using food. You need to ignite or reignite your passions, so you can transition from a life in which you are surviving to a life in which you are *thriving*.

If you've been knee-deep in Sugar for a long time, then it might feel challenging, even scary, to think about where you can find nourishment elsewhere in your life. It can be particularly scary because it requires a level of vulnerability to try new things and step outside your comfort zone. But, as best-selling author Neale Donald Walsch said, "Life begins at the end of your comfort zone." It's time to take that leap of faith into your new life.

Think back to a time you can remember doing something or connecting with someone and you feeling a sense of excitement or fulfillment. Maybe you used to love to paint or take long walks in the park. Perhaps you loved going to concerts or taking road trips. Think about those joyous and connected moments and let this be your launching pad. If you pay close attention to your life without Sugar, little joyful feelings will start to pop up: a puppy on the street, the smell after it rains, your favorite TV show, your best friend's laughter. Start to make note of the little joys, and they will snowball into bigger joys.

Also reflect on emotions and experiences you want to participate in more fully, such as love, excitement, or peace, and think about ways in which you can invite them in: joining a gardening club, learning how to square dance, writing short stories, dating, discovering astrology, spending more time with your children. The list goes on and on. What's most important is that you place a priority on creating positive experiences and interests. These will nourish your spirit and bring you joy, making it less likely you'll be tempted to turn back to Sugar.

You'll need to schedule time in your calendar for this one or have a reminder on your phone so you can remember to practice things that bring you joy.

With a dash of self-love

We've talked so much about the rehabilitation of your relationship with food. But how will you heal the relationship with *yourself*? How will you ever be able to practice self-love and build back your self-esteem? Those can seem like impossible concepts when you haven't experienced them . . . maybe ever.

Lucky for us, self-love and self-esteem are buy-one-get-both action steps. Every time you turn to Sugar, your light gets dimmed. And each time you succumb to the pull, the negative voice in your head concludes, once again, that you'll never be able to do this, that you're doomed, a failure. Even worse, after multiple transgressions, it may conclude you're unlovable or unworthy.

Though it may not have been accomplished perfectly, you made the commitment in the Sacred Vow to stay this course—to not cut and run, regardless of how much you want to, how sexy that sprinkled cupcake looks, or how loud the committee in your mind is screaming at you.

Here's the secret recipe: **You create self-love and build self-esteem by being kind to and acting estimably toward yourself.** It's accomplished by doing what you say you're going to do, by taking the harder route and using a Right Now Skill when numbing with Sugar would be so much easier, by prepping your lunch even though you're exhausted, by saying a firm no thank-you when you're offered the cookies at the Christmas party for the fifth time. Every single one of these small actions makes a deposit into your depleted bank account of self-love and esteem.

Every day that you show up for yourself—both in feeling and in action—in the name of the life you know you deserve is a day that you make amends to yourself for the days you did not. And before you know it, that committee in your mind will be quieter and quieter. Better yet, it will turn into a new voice, one that cheers you on for how far you've come, how amazing you are, and how bright the path ahead is.

Your Sacred Vow is the alpha and the omega. By honoring it, you can navigate and flourish within your new relationship. With patience, trust, and commitment, you'll be entering a whole new world where Sugar, Flour, and compulsive dieting are no longer your master, the exhaustion of self-hate off your back.

I could not be more excited for you to begin to be the commander of your new life—to reclaim the power and light you've lost. I cannot wait to see who you become and how that will change your life and the world around you. Welcome to your new life and your very best you.

Postscript: A Love Letter from Me

Even though I don't know you, I love you. I love you because you are one of the bravest people I know. And I love you because we are family.

Do you even understand how hard it is to pick up a book called *Breaking Up with Sugar*? To read it, and to follow at least some of its suggestions? That takes courage that most rarely exhibit. Despite all the voices in your head telling you not to and all evidence to the contrary, you mustered the willingness for another go-round with your relationship with food. *You* did that. Which means that you are really something. Take that in. You picked this book up. You finished it. You chose *yourself* over the ease of the familiar pattern you've been living in.

I don't know if these are the exact right words for it—warrior, champion, rock star, diva, survivor, star—but you are extraordinary, to say the least. I know what the words *aren't*: loser, failure, too fat, untreatable, commitment-phobic, unlovable, broken—all those words you were regularly using before we met. Which, by the way, you weren't then, either. If you're still holding on to the belief that you are damaged goods, that you can't commit to this, that you're a hopeless case, I beg you to kick it to the curb—or at least call it out for the liar it is.

Because, as I've told you a trillion times throughout this book, times are going to get tough—life will get lifey—and I want you to remember how far you've come, just by reading a book! Imagine what you are capable of as your new relationships flourish. I'm a part of your Power

Circle now, and I hope you'll carry my voice with you for years to come. You have my complete and total support, and with that comes my fierce love and commitments.

And we need to say, right now, in this moment, out loud, that you are stronger than you know. You are the kind of person who boldly chooses the hard path. You may not know that, so it needs to be emphasized, shouted from the rooftops. I want you to take all the light and all the hope you've cultivated—even if you're scared of it. Put these in a bottle to open and revel in when you need it most.

We all reach these pivotal moments in life when there are two roads presented to us. We can choose to stay the way we are or take the hard and unfamiliar route. I call those moments my "grow or die," or GOD moments. Those are the times I have had to dig deeper, try harder, and get back up again—and each and every time, I have become stronger for it. It is what has given me back my spirit after Sugar and dieting ravaged it and claimed it for their own.

I hope this is a GOD moment for you. I want this to be the time you bravely choose the unknown path—the one that looks harder and scarier, but gives you back the spirit that's been stolen from you and makes you proud of your own strength and resilience.

Whether you realize it or not, life, spirit, the universe—whatever you want to call this flow we are in—is tapping you on the shoulder and saying, *Now is the time.* That's what happened to you here—a little GOD, a little grace—and I never want you to forget that. Ever.

And more than that, I want you to continue on your journey. Maybe you've taken one step in the direction of your freedom, maybe five, or maybe you're all in. The seeds of possibility have been planted, and if you tend to them, *they will grow.* You have no idea what a vibrant and fulfilling life awaits you post-breakup. A world where you are deeply committed to nurturing this new life of yours and this new relationship with yourself. It's bigger and brighter than you could ever imagine. Pinky swear.

May this breakup be the beginning of the healing from your diet drama and trauma. May this breakup be the reclaiming of the truth of who you really are, helping you take back all that's been stolen from you. May this breakup be the beginning of so many new and brave adventures. You have so much light to shine, so much to offer the world and to help inspire it. I'm so excited to see where you take this, my friend.

Xxx,

Milly

PS: I always want to know what you're up to and what you're thinking about, and I want you to know the same about me. Right now, I want to know what is inspiring you. Go to mybreakupwithsugar.com and share your personal commitment statement with me and your new family of Breakup Buddies! From there, you'll get to connect with your very best friends you don't know yet, find more resources for your new life, be up-to-date on upcoming events, and so much more. See you there!

Skills Calling Card

Skill to Date This Week: *(see the Skills in the following pages)*

Right-Now Skills

1. _____
2. _____
3. _____

Long-Lasting Skills

1. _____
2. _____
3. _____

Do you like this skill?   Do you want to date   Should this skill go into
                                 this skill again?   your toolbox?

☐ yes   ☐ no   ☐ yes   ☐ no   ☐ yes   ☐ no

Right-Now Skills

Distract when you're alone

Get into a new book or TV show

Get crafty

Take a walk outside

Call up a friend

Create your own: _____

Distract when you're with other people

Go to the bathroom/ take a break

Splash face with cold water

Imagine coping with the situation effectively

Imagine you are somewhere else

Create your own: _____

Self-Soothe Skills

Take a hot shower or bath

Use incense or scented diffuser

Listen to music

Snuggle with your pet

Create your own:_____

Emergency Skills

Deep Breathing

Progressive muscle relaxation

Use an ice pack

Long-Lasting Skills

Connection
Join a club

Go to a religious service

Get in touch with family or friends

Go to a self-help meeting

Create your own:_____

Prayer & Gratitude
Write Gratitude Journal

Do silent prayer

Say a mantra to yourself

Go to a religious service

Create your own:_____

Meditation
Do a meditation on your phone app

Focus on your breath

Focus on one of your senses

Do a walking meditation

Create your own:_____

Body and Movement
Take a walk

Take an exercise class

Play a sport

Go for a gentle hike

Create your own:_____

Relationship Rebuild Recipes

BREAKFAST CONCEPTS (choose one a day)

2 servings Protein + 1 serving Carbohydrate + 1 serving Fruit or Fat

2 servings Protein + 2 servings Carbohydrate

3 servings Protein + 1 serving Carbohydrate or Fruit

Veggies optional at every breakfast

LUNCH & DINNER CONCEPTS (choose two a day)

3–5 servings Protein + 1 serving Carbohydrate + 1 serving Fat
    + Veggies*

3 servings Protein + 1–2 servings Carbohydrate + 1 serving
    Fat + Veggies*

3–5 servings Protein + 2 servings Fat + Veggies*

SNACK CONCEPTS (choose one a day)

2 servings Protein + 1 serving Fruit/ Veggies*

2 servings Fat + Veggies*

2 servings Protein + 1 serving Carbohydrate

Food Breakdown

*VEGETABLES

A serving of vegetables is typically three cups raw or two cups cooked. But let's be honest, your relationship with food didn't get dysfunctional because of too many veggies, so if you want a little more, go on with your bad self.

PROTEIN CHOICES

Not all protein choices are created equal! Remember to be calorie conscious not calorie counting.

Each Protein listed below is 1 serving

Have 1 ounce of:
Veal
Beef
Pork
Lamb
Dark-meat chicken
Sausage (Sugar-free)
Tofu/Tempeh
Salmon
Cheese

Have 2 ounces of:
Turkey
Tuna
White-meat chicken
Fish/Shellfish (not salmon)
Cold cuts (Sugar-free)

Here are some other protein measurements that might come in handy:
3 egg whites (¼ cup)
½ ounce seeds (raw and unsalted)
½ cup edamame in pods
⅓ cup shelled edamame
⅓ cup cooked beans or legumes (can be used as a carb or
    protein—dealer's choice)
½ cup 1 percent cottage cheese
½ cup 1–2 percent plain yogurt
8 ounces 1 percent or skim milk
¼ cup part-skim ricotta cheese

½ cup meatless crumbles

1 Laughing Cow wedge (not Light)

1 whole egg

1 tablespoon nut butter

½ ounce nuts (raw, unsalted)

½ Gardenburger veggie burger

CARBOHYDRATE CHOICES

Each Carbohydrate listed below is 1 serving

1 slice Ezekiel bread*

1 Ezekiel wrap*

*Contains sprouted whole grain and does not contain flour. It can be found in the freezer aisle of the grocery store.

½ **cup COOKED** (⅓ **cup dry; 1 ounce dry**)

Oatmeal

Oat bran

Rice (no white, red, or yellow)

Quinoa

Here are some other carbohydrate measurements that might come in handy:

4 ounces cooked potato

4 ounces cooked sweet potato

4 ounces cooked yams

3 ounces cooked yucca

1 ear corn

1 cup peas

4 tablespoons (¼ cup) hummus

4 ounces cooked winter squash (acorn, butternut, Hubbard, pumpkin, spaghetti, delicata)

2–3 rice cakes (brown rice only; about 90–120 calories)

2 Wasa crackers (no sesame, sourdough, or light)

12 Mary's Gone Crackers

⅓ cup cooked beans or legumes (can be used as a carb or
   protein—dealer's choice)

FRUIT CHOICES

Most Fruit servings are 1 whole fruit or 6 ounces

These are fruits that are higher in calorie and sugar content. My
recommendation is to eat these in 3-ounce portions:

Acai

Banana (½ medium banana)

Figs

Grapes

Mango

Papaya

Pineapple

Pomegranate

FAT CHOICES

Each Fat listed below is 1 serving

1 tablespoon butter

2 tablespoons reduced-fat butter or margarine

1 tablespoon oil

1 tablespoon mayonnaise

3 tablespoons guacamole

3 tablespoons sour cream

1 tablespoon tahini

2 tablespoons cream cheese

15 olives

⅓ medium avocado (2 ounces)

1 tablespoon (½ ounce) nuts and seeds (almonds, Brazil nuts,
   butternuts, cashews, chia, flax, hazelnuts, hemp, macadamia nuts,
   peanuts, pecans, pine nuts, pumpkin seeds, pistachios, sesame
   seeds, soy nuts, squash seeds, sunflower seeds, walnuts)

Relationship Rebuild Recipes

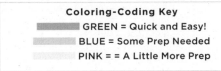

All recipes below indicate one serving size for the designated meal or snack.

BREAKFAST RECIPES

2 servings Protein + 1 serving Carbohydrate + 1 serving Fruit or Fat

QUICK AND EASY

Cottage Cheese Tartine (Vegetarian)	Spread 1 cup 1% cottage cheese on top of 1 piece toasted Ezekiel bread. Top with ½ medium banana (3 ounces) or ¾ cup sliced strawberries. Sprinkle with cinnamon.
Breakfast on the Run (Vegan)	Spread 2 tablespoons nut butter on top of 1 piece toasted Ezekiel bread. Top with ½ medium banana (3 ounces), sliced.
Breakfast at the Diner	Order 2 eggs scrambled (with optional veggies added), ½ cup cooked oatmeal, and 1 fruit serving.
Breakfast at Starbucks	Choose either: Sous Vide Egg Bites: Bacon & Gruyere or Sous Vide Egg Bites: Egg White and Red Pepper + ½ medium banana (3 ounces) or 1 packet avocado spread

SOME PREP NEEDED

Eggs and Berries on Toast (Vegetarian)	2 eggs (cooked any way you want) + 1 slice toasted Ezekiel bread + ¾ cup mixed berries OR 1 tablespoon butter (for toast)
Yogurt Parfait (Vegetarian)	½ cup 2% unsweetened Greek yogurt + dash vanilla extract with ½ cup cooked quinoa + 4 tablespoons unsweetened raw coconut flakes, 1 tablespoon slivered almonds, ½ cup mixed berries. Mix together and enjoy!
Morning Apple Pie Bowl (Vegetarian)	In a bowl, mix ½ cup cooked oatmeal (⅓ cup dry) with ½ cup 2% unsweetened Greek yogurt. Sprinkle with cinnamon or apple pie spice. Top with 1 tablespoon chopped almonds and 1 sliced medium apple.
Nutter Butter Bowl (Vegan)	In a bowl, combine ½ cup cooked oatmeal (⅓ cup dry), ½ medium banana (3 ounces), 2 tablespoons natural almond butter, and 2 tablespoons unsweetened almond milk. Microwave for 1 minute and enjoy!

A LITTLE MORE PREP

Ricotta and Mushroom Tartine (national breakfast of France!)	⅛ cup sliced cremini or favorite small mushroom ⅛ cup sliced onions ½ cup part-skim ricotta cheese ½ teaspoon lemon zest or fresh chives (optional) 1 slice Ezekiel bread, toasted Heat a nonstick pan over medium heat. Spray with cooking spray. Add the mushrooms and onions, adding spray if needed and stirring occasionally, until most of the liquid is absorbed, 5 minutes. Mix the ricotta and lemon zest (if using) in a small bowl. Spread the ricotta on top of the toasted Ezekiel bread. Top with the mushrooms and onions. Eat with fruit of your choice.
Taco Skillet Frittata	4 ounces cooked sweet potato ¼ tablespoon cumin ⅛ teaspoon salt ⅛ cup diced onion ⅛ cup diced bell pepper ½ cup meatless crumbles Chili powder, to taste 3 egg whites ⅓ medium avocado (2 ounces), diced Fresh cilantro Heat a nonstick pan over medium-high heat. Spray with cooking spray. Add the sweet potato, cumin, and salt. Cook for 5 minutes, stirring occasionally. Add the diced onion and bell pepper. Cook for 5 minutes. Add the meatless crumbles and cook for another 5 minutes. Add chili powder. Add the egg whites to the pan and mix them into the cooked crumbles mixture. Let the mixture cook, covered, until set, 2 to 3 minutes. To serve, top with the avocado and cilantro.
Bacon, Eggs, and Avocado Quesadilla	Cook 3 egg whites. Place in an Ezekiel wrap and add 1 ounce turkey bacon or Canadian bacon and ⅓ medium avocado (2 ounces), sliced. Wrap. Heat in a pan until crispy.

BREAKFAST

2 servings Protein + 2 servings Carbohydrate

QUICK AND EASY

Grilled Cheese (Vegetarian)	Melt 2 ounces cheese between 2 pieces toasted Ezekiel bread.

PB 2 GO (Vegan)	Spread 2 tablespoons almond butter over 2 pieces toasted Ezekiel bread.
Sweet PotaEggo (Vegetarian)	Place 2 over-easy eggs on top of 8 ounces cooked sweet potato.
Cottage Cup (Vegetarian)	Mix together 1 cup 1% cottage cheese, ½ sliced medium banana (3 ounces), and 7 walnut halves.

BREAKFAST

3 servings Protein + 1 serving Carbohydrate or Fruit

SOME PREP NEEDED

Breakfast in a Minute MUG (Vegetarian)	In a mug, combine 2 eggs, 1 ounce feta cheese, ½ cup cooked oatmeal (⅓ cup dry), spinach, and diced red peppers and onions. Microwave for 90 seconds.
Overnight Chia Pudding Breakfast (Vegetarian)	In a mason jar, mix 2 tablespoons chia seeds, ½ cup 2% yogurt, ½ cup cooked quinoa or brown rice, and a dash of vanilla. Make in the evening, refrigerate, and enjoy in the morning.
Egg Muffins	Preheat the oven to 350°F. Beat 2 eggs and mix with 2 ounces deli turkey. Pour into muffin tins and bake for 10 minutes. Enjoy with a slice of toasted Ezekiel bread on the side.

LUNCH & DINNER

3 to 5 servings Protein + 1 serving Carbohydrate + 1 serving Fat + Veggies*

QUICK AND EASY

Tuna Tortilla	Mix 6 ounces all-white tuna (packed in water and drained) with 1 tablespoon mayo and 2 tablespoons 2% Greek yogurt. Spread on 1 Ezekiel wrap, add lettuce and tomato, and fold in half.
Lunch/Dinner from Chipotle (Or make at home!): Burrito Bowl with Lettuce	Made with a base of lettuce, 6 ounces chopped chicken (approximately 1 scoop at Chipotle), ⅓ cup black beans (approximately 1 scoop), and 6 to 8 ounces of fajita vegetables (approximately 1 scoop). Get 3 tablespoons guacamole on the side to top off the salad!
Lunch/Dinner from Panera	Greek with Chicken Salad

SOME PREP NEEDED

Egg (Vegetarian) or Tofu (Vegan) Wrap	½ cup chopped veggies Salt and pepper 3 eggs or 3 ounces pressed firm tofu 1 Ezekiel wrap ⅓ medium avocado (2 ounces) Heat a nonstick pan over medium-high heat. Spray with cooking spray. Add ½ cup raw chopped vegetables, season with salt and pepper, and cook for 3 to 5 minutes, until vegetables soften. In a small bowl, scramble 3 eggs. Add the eggs to the vegetables. Add the avocado. Wrap it all up in 1 Ezekiel wrap and enjoy.
Power Potato	Fill a small (4-ounce) baked sweet potato with ¾ cup chopped broccoli, 8 ounces grilled white-meat chicken, and 1 tablespoon melted butter. Sprinkle with chives.
Gardenburger Stacks (Vegetarian)	Cook 2 Gardenburger veggie burgers according to package instructions. Place each burger on one side of an open-faced Ezekiel bun. Pile each with thick tomato slices and lettuce leaves and add grilled, baked, or sautéed sliced portobello mushrooms. Drizzle each stack with 1 tablespoon no-Sugar dressing.
Greek Spinach Sensation (Vegetarian)	In a large bowl, toss together spinach leaves, chopped cucumbers, ⅔ cup chickpeas or any bean, sliced tomatoes, 2 ounces tofu, 1 to 2 ounces feta cheese, 5 sliced black olives. and 1 tablespoon no-Sugar Greek dressing with 1 to 2 tablespoons balsamic vinegar.
Stuffed Lettuce Wraps	4 Bibb lettuce wraps ¼ cup (4 tablespoons) hummus 8 ounces deli turkey 1 hard-boiled egg 4 ounces chopped onion Salt and pepper 4 ounces crunchy vegetables (e.g., green or red bell pepper) 1 tablespoon no-Sugar dressing Line each of the lettuce wraps with 1 tablespoon of hummus. Fill each hummus-lined Bibb lettuce leaf with a total of 2 ounces chopped deli turkey. Chop up one hard-boiled egg. Mix the chopped egg, tomato, and onion together. Add chopped egg, onion, and tomato mixture to each Bibb lettuce wrap. Season to taste with salt and pepper. Serve with crunchy vegetables like green and red pepper on the side and dip them into 1 tablespoon of your favorite no-Sugar dressing.
Soft Taco Tuesday (Vegetarian)	1½ cups Morningstar Farms meatless crumbles ½ cup chopped tomatoes ½ cup chopped or shredded lettuce 1 Ezekiel wrap

	⅓ cup salsa 3 tablespoons sour cream ¼ cup shredded Mexican cheese Cook the meatless crumbles in a nonstick pan over medium heat. Add the tomatoes and shredded lettuce. Wrap the mixture in the wrap. Mix together the salsa and sour cream. To serve, top the wrap with the salsa mixture and shredded cheese. Note: Taco mixture may spill over and not all fit in your wrap. That's ok. Be sure to scoop it up and eat taco salad with your salsa.
Open-faced Burger with Salad	Heat a grill pan over medium-high heat on the stove. Pre-season a 3- to 4-ounce hamburger patty with a total of ½ teaspoon total garlic salt split between both sides of the burger. Place the burger on the heated pan. Leave the burger alone for 3 minutes. Flip the burger and continue cooking for another 4 to 5 minutes to allow the other side to brown. Cook the burger until it reaches 160°F on a meat thermometer. Place on top of 1 slice toasted Ezekiel bread with tomato slices, ⅓ sliced avocado (2 ounces), and 1 ounce cheese. Serve with a side salad with 1 tablespoon of your favorite no-Sugar dressing.
Easy Roast Chicken Dinner	Serve 6 to 8 ounces white meat (3 to 5 ounces if dark) from a store-bought rotisserie chicken with ¾ cup steamed veggies and a small cooked sweet potato (4 ounces), topped with 1 tablespoon melted butter.

A LITTLE MORE PREP

Vegetarian Rancheros	¼ cup onion ½ teaspoon chili powder ½ teaspoon cumin ½ teaspoon oregano ⅓ cup tomato sauce ⅓ cup refried beans 2 ounces firm tofu Juice of ½ lime 1 Ezekiel wrap 1 teaspoon cilantro ¼ cup chopped tomato 3 tablespoons sour cream Heat a skillet over medium heat. Spray with cooking spray. Add the onion, chili powder, cumin, and oregano and cook for 2 to 3 minutes. Stir in the tomato sauce, beans, tofu, and lime juice. Sauté for 5 minutes. Spread the mixture on top of the wrap. Top with cilantro, tomatoes, and sour cream.
Sausage and Peppers	3 to 5 ounces Aidells brand chicken sausage, chopped into chunks ½ onion, chopped 1 green bell pepper, chopped ½ to 1 garlic clove, minced

	Salt and pepper ½ cup chicken broth ½ cup cooked quinoa or brown rice Up to 1 tablespoon chopped parsley for serving 3 tablespoons sour cream or ⅓ medium avocado (2 ounces), sliced Heat a pan over medium heat and spray with cooking spray. Cook the sausage until golden, about 2 minutes. Add the onion, green pepper, garlic, and salt and pepper. Cook for 2 to 3 more minutes. Add the broth and bring to a gentle simmer. Pour all of it over the quinoa or brown rice. Top with the sour cream.
White Pizza (Vegetarian)	Ezekiel tortilla ½ cup part-skim ricotta cheese ¼ cup shredded part-skim mozzarella cheese 1 tablespoon shredded Parmesan cheese Garlic powder, to taste Italian seasoning, to taste Chopped spinach Salt and pepper 2 cups mixed greens 1 tablespoon of your favorite Sugar-free dressing Preheat the oven to 350°F. Lightly spray the wrap with olive oil spray and bake for 5 minutes. In a bowl, combine the ricotta, mozzarella, Parmesan, garlic powder, and Italian seasoning. Spread the cheese mixture over the wrap and top with chopped spinach (alternative approach: Mix the chopped spinach into cheese mixture, then spread the cheese and spinach mixture onto the wrap). Finish with a sprinkle of salt and pepper. Bake for 20 to 25 minutes. Serve with a side of 2 cups mixed greens and 1 tablespoon of your favorite Sugar-free dressing.
Try-a-Stir-fry (Vegan)	3 to 5 ounces extra-firm tofu, cubed 8 ounces of frozen stir-fry vegetables, cooked according to manufacturer's instructions 1 tablespoon soy sauce 1 tablespoon toasted sesame oil ½ cup cooked brown rice Spray pan with cooking spray and heat over medium-high heat. Arrange the tofu in a single layer in the hot pan, and let it sear/cook for 1 minute. Then stir-fry tofu for another minute (Note: When stir-frying tofu, heat the tofu to soften it, not pan-fry. You may not see browning). Next, stir in the veggies, add the soy sauce, toasted sesame oil, and cooked brown rice. Cook all together for another 3 to 4 minutes. Plate it and enjoy!

LUNCH & DINNER

3 servings Protein + 1 to 2 servings Carbohydrate + 1 serving Fat + Veggies*

QUICK AND EASY

Sandwich on the Run	Make a sandwich with 2 pieces toasted Ezekiel bread, 6 ounces deli turkey, and 1 tablespoon mayonnaise. Add lettuce, tomato, salt, and pepper and you're out the door.
Lunch/Dinner at American-fare restaurant	Order a 3-egg-white omelet cooked with 2 ounces turkey/ham/chicken, chopped spinach, mushrooms, and 1 ounce cheese. Add ½ cup salsa on the side with ⅓ medium avocado (2 ounces), sliced. Eat with a side of 4 ounces of potato.

SOME PREP NEEDED

Burrit-No-Bowl	In a bowl, combine 6 ounces chopped, cooked white-meat chicken breast, ⅓ to ⅔ cup rice and beans combo, ⅓ medium avocado (2 ounces) sliced, and chopped tomato.
Cheesy Spuds and Eggs (Vegetarian)	Cook 1 cup egg whites in a nonstick pan. Separately cook a 4- to 6-ounce potato in the microwave. Break the baked potato open, load in the cooked egg whites, and melt 1 ounce cheese on top with either 1 tablespoon butter or 3 tablespoons sour cream and chopped chives.
Soup and Sandwich	Heat 1 can Progresso Light Chicken and Wild Rice Soup. Add ⅓ medium avocado. Serve with 1 piece toasted Ezekiel bread toasted in the oven with 1 slice cheese.

A LITTLE MORE PREP

Pizzzzalicious	Preheat oven to 350°F. Bake 1 Ezekiel wrap for 5 minutes. Mix ½ cup low-fat or 1% cottage cheese with ⅓ cup tomato sauce and spread over the baked wrap. Top with ¼ cup part-skim shredded mozzarella cheese, 1 ounce cooked ground beef (or 2 ounces lean ground chicken), and finely chopped vegetables (cooked or raw). Bake for 8 to 10 minutes. Serve with a side of 2 cups mixed greens and 1 tablespoon of your favorite Sugar-free dressing.
Fish Dish	1 6-ounce tilapia filet (or fish of your choice) 1 tablespoon melted butter or olive oil 1 tablespoon lemon juice ½ teaspoon garlic powder

Salt and pepper
1 tablespoon capers, drained
⅛ teaspoon oregano
Dash of paprika
1 tablespon olive oil
1 teaspoon sesame seeds
1 12-ounce bag of steamed vegetables
½ cup cooked brown rice

Preheat oven to 400°F.
To bake: Prepare a fresh piece of 6-ounce tilapia (or fish of your choice): grill, bake, broil, or poach.
To bake: Place tilapia in an ungreased 8-inch square baking dish. In a small bowl, combine the melted butter, lemon juice, garlic powder, and salt; pour over the fillet. Sprinkle with capers, oregano, and paprika. Bake, uncovered, for 10 to 15 minutes or until the fish flakes easily with a fork.
To broil: Preheat the broiler, line a broiler pan with foil, and coat it with nonstick spray. Rub a total of 1 tablespoon extra-virgin olive oil into both sides of the fillet, season with a dash of salt and pepper on both sides. Place the tilapia under the broiler, about 4 inches from the heat, and broil for 4 minutes. Carefully turn the fish over and broil for an additional 4 minutes.
Cook steamed vegetables according to package instructions.
Plate the fish with the cooked brown rice and vegetables.

LUNCH & DINNER

3 to 5 servings Protein + 2 servings Fat + Veggies*

SOME PREP NEEDED

Shrimp Salad	In a large bowl, combine chopped romaine lettuce, 6 to 8 ounces chopped and cooked jumbo shrimp, 1 sliced hard-boiled egg, cherry tomatoes, and chopped cucumber. Toss with 2 tablespoons regular-fat, no-Sugar blue cheese dressing.
HamBLEU burger	Heat a grill pan over medium-high heat on the stove. Pre-season a 3- to 5-ounce hamburger patty with a total of ½ teaspoon garlic salt on both sides of the patty. Place the burger on the heated pan. Leave the burger alone for 3 minutes. Flip the burger and continue cooking for another 4 to 5 minutes to allow the other side to brown. Cook the burger until it reaches 160°F on a meat thermometer. Preheat the oven to 450°F. Wipe the portobello mushroom caps with paper towels. Remove the stems. Line a baking sheet with aluminum foil and arrange the mushroom cap gills-side up in one layer on top of the foil. Sprinkle with salt and pepper.

	Roast mushrooms in the oven until they are lightly browned, 10 to 12 minutes, depending on the crispiness you prefer (Note: Roasting portobello mushrooms will give the mushroom a crispy exterior—similar to toasting a bun). Remove the mushroom bun from the oven. Place the burger between 2 large cooked portobello mushroom "buns." Drizzle with 2 tablespoons of regular-fat, no-Sugar blue cheese dressing.
The Big Salad	In a large bowl, toss lettuce, 1 ounce goat cheese, 1 tablespoon chopped nuts, and vegetables of your choice. Top with a 3-ounce piece of baked or grilled salmon and drizzle with 1 tablespoon no-Sugar dressing.
PortoBleuVeggie Burger (Vegetarian)	Cook 2 Morningstar Farms Grillers veggie burgers according to package instructions. Preheat the oven to 450°F. Wipe the portobello mushroom caps with paper towels. Remove the stems. Line a baking sheet with aluminum foil and arrange the mushroom caps gills-side up in one layer on top of the foil. Sprinkle with salt and pepper. Roast mushrooms in the oven until they are lightly browned, 10 to 12 minutes, depending on the crispiness you prefer (Note: Roasting portobello mushrooms will give the mushroom a crispy exterior—similar to toasting a bun). Remove the mushroom buns from the oven. Place between 2 cooked portobello mushroom "buns" (or serve open-faced). Drizzle with 2 tablespoons regular-fat, no-Sugar blue cheese dressing.
Cauli-It-EASY Fried Rice (Vegetarian)	1 12-ounce bag Green Giant Riced Veggies Cauliflower Medley, cooked according to package instructions, or cooked cauliflower rice with cooked chopped veggies of your choice 1 to 2 tablespoons soy sauce 2 whole eggs plus ½ cup egg whites 2 tablespoons toasted sesame oil Heat a skillet over medium heat. Spray with cooking spray, add the cooked cauliflower medley and soy sauce, and heat for 5 minutes. Add the eggs and egg whites and cook for 4 to 5 minutes, until egg is cooked within rice mixture. Stir in the sesame oil and cook for another 1 to 2 minutes to toss and heat oil all the way through the rice.
Zoodle Bolognese	Heat a nonstick skillet with 1 tablespoon oil over medium heat until hot. Add 3 to 5 ounces lean ground beef and cook 3 to 4 minutes, breaking beef into ½-inch crumbles and stirring occasionally until meat is browned and heated through. Add ½ cup tomato sauce to browned beef and cook for 1 minute. Add 8 ounces (1 cup) zoodles (about 1 zucchini; see Note) and another ½ cup tomato sauce. Reduce heat to low and cook for another 5 to 10 minutes. Top with 3 tablespoons sour cream for serving.

Note: For best results, place the zoodles in a colander over the sink and toss with 3 dashes of salt. Let them sit for 30 minutes. The salt will bring out the water. After half an hour, squeeze the zoodles gently to release some additional water. Stir fry them for 5 minutes over medium-high heat.

A LITTLE MORE PREP

Spicy Cashew Stir-fry (Vegetarian)	One 6 to 8-ounce bag frozen stir-fry vegetables or fresh chopped carrots, broccoli, red bell pepper, and onion ⅓ cup vegetable broth 2 tablespoons soy sauce 1 to 2 tablespoons chili garlic sauce 1 teaspoon grated fresh ginger (optional) 3 ounces raw cashews 2 tablespoons toasted sesame oil In a large skillet over medium-high heat, cook the vegetables with the broth, soy sauce, chili garlic sauce, and ginger (if using). If using frozen veggies, cook according to package instructions. If cooking fresh veggies, cook until the onions just begin to soften, 3 to 5 minutes. Add the cashews and toss with the sesame oil.
Stuffed Pepper of Goodness	2 green bell peppers Salt ½ onion, chopped 5 ounces mushrooms, chopped 1 tomato, chopped 4 ounces ground beef 1 ounce shredded cheese 2 cups mixed greens 2 tablespoons of your favorite Sugar-free dressing Preheat the oven to 350°F. Cut off the tops of the peppers, reserving them, and discard the seeds and membranes. Boil peppers for 5 minutes and invert to drain. Lightly salt the inside of peppers. Chop up reserved pepper tops and combine with onion, mushroom, and tomato. Heat a large nonstick skillet over medium heat until hot. Add ground beef and pepper mixture. Cook 3 to 4 minutes, breaking beef into ½-inch crumbles and stirring occasionally. Cook until meat is browned and heated through. Divide beef mixture evenly among peppers and top with the shredded cheese. Bake in 350°F oven for 30 minutes, until instant-read thermometer inserted into center of beef mixture registers 160° F and bell peppers are tender. Serve with mixed greens and 2 tablespoons of your favorite Sugar-free dressing.

SNACK

2 servings Protein + 1 serving Fruit/ Vegetables*

QUICK AND EASY

Grab and Go (Vegan)	One Basix, Primal Kitchen, or Raw Rev Glo brand protein bar* + 1 serving fruit (optional) *Protein bars can be triggering for some. Please use them responsibly—if you start to obsess about them or eat too many, they may not be a food that works for you. Please note: All Breaking Up with Sugar–approved protein bars must contain: • 3 grams of sugar or less—including sugar alcohols (e.g., erythritol) • 250 calories or less • 11 grams protein or more • 5 grams fiber or more
Cinnamon-Apple Yogurt (Vegetarian)	Add 6 ounces chopped apple to 1 cup unsweetened 2% Greek yogurt and sprinkle with cinnamon.
Veggies and Yogurt Dip (Vegetarian)	Combine 1 cup unsweetened 2% Greek yogurt with garlic or onion powder and herbs. Serve as a dip with 6 ounces cut vegetables, such as carrots, celery sticks, or peppers.
Yogurt and Berries (Vegetarian)	Mix 1 cup 2% unsweetened yogurt with ¾ cup sliced strawberries.
Banana and Nuts (Vegan)	Slice ½ medium banana (3 ounces). Crush up 1 ounce nuts (any kind!) in a bag. Press the banana slices into the crushed nuts.
Protein and Grapes (Vegetarian)	2 part-skim mozzarella cheese sticks (or 1 ounce nuts) + ¾ cup grapes
Apple Slice Sandwich (Vegan)	Slice 1 apple, then spread 2 tablespoons almond butter on the slices. Put two together to make sandwiches.
Tomato and Mozzarella Sandwich (Vegetarian)	Slice up 1 beefsteak tomato. Place 2 ounces sliced part-skim mozzarella cheese and fresh basil between tomato slices. Drizzle with 1 to 2 tablespoons balsamic vinegar. Add fresh ground pepper to taste.

SOME PREP NEEDED

Cucumber Bites (Vegetarian)	Slice 1 small cucumber into coins. Top coins with 2 hard-boiled eggs, sliced. Sprinkle with salt and pepper to taste.

SNACK

2 servings Fat + Vegetables*

QUICK AND EASY

Veggies and Dressing (Vegan or Vegetarian)	Dip 1 cup sliced peppers into 2 tablespoons no-Sugar salad dressing.
Veggies with Guac (Vegan)	6 tablespoons guacamole + 6 ounces carrot sticks, bell pepper slices, cucumber coins, or jicama sticks
Snack on the Go (Vegan)	Two 100-calorie packs raw nuts (usually walnuts or almonds). Eat with 6 ounces baby carrots or vegetable of your choice.

SOME PREP NEEDED

Avocado and Tomato Salad (Vegan)	Slice ⅓ medium avocado (2 ounces) and 1 tomato. Arrange avocado on top of tomato slices. Add 1 tablespoon olive oil or no-Sugar dressing and sprinkle with salt and pepper.

SNACK

2 servings Protein + 1 serving Carbohydrate

QUICK AND EASY

Cinnamon Oatmeal (Vegetarian)	Mix ½ cup cooked oatmeal (⅓ cup dry) with ½ cup part-skim ricotta cheese and sprinkle with cinnamon.
Turkey and Crackers	4 ounces sliced turkey with 12 Mary's Gone Crackers
Peanut or Almond Butter Toast (Vegan)	Spread 2 tablespoons almond or peanut butter over 1 piece toasted Ezekiel bread.
Cheese and Crackers (Vegetarian)	Spread 2 Laughing Cow cheese wedges on 2 Wasa crackers.

Turkey and Cheese Wrap	Place 2 ounces turkey and 1 ounce cheese on an Ezekiel wrap or toast.
Chicken and Hummus	Top 4 ounces grilled white-meat chicken with 100-calorie hummus individual pack (or 4 tablespoons).

Acknowledgments

Acknowledgments? Not quite. More like the declaration of my appreciation from the bottom of my heart and soul to the people who have helped make this book a reality. If you know me well, you know I could write a standalone book expressing my gratitude—so believe it or not, I'm keeping it brief.

I am profoundly grateful to my agent, now one of my truest and closest friends, Stephanie Tade, who saw past a therapist without a platform right to my pure essence and how badly I want to help people. Thank you for your wisdom, your intuition and your love. The absolute same can be said for the incredible team at Avery: Thank you to my editor, "Saint Lucia" Watson, and Avery's publisher, Megan Newman, who have taken this big leap with me with excitement and care. Cartwheels of love and gratitude to the rest of the team, whose diligence and talent blows me out of the water and who fostered an unknown love for Tibetan singing bowls when taking me on: Anne Kosmoski, Sara Johnson, Allyssa Fortunato, Farin Schlussel, Rachel Dugan, Suzy Swartz, and Lindsay Gordon. And to PR queen Heidi Krupp, who has been rooting me on since back in the day. Thank you to my dear friend Michelle Garside, for always seeing me wholly and believing in me enough to introduce me to Stephanie, where the ball really got rolling.

Thank you to Nikki Glantz for her contributing genius to this idea—fiercely providing flexible, honest, hilarious, and supportive vibes throughout every incarnation of this book over the last six years. Thank you to Marty and Michele Lerner, who have become family, for their undying support and for letting Nikki and I hijack their house on more occasions than I can count.

A special and separate thank-you to Alexandra Wilt, my writing partner and researcher extraordinaire, who has a constant notes page ready when I scream out a thought and always said yes, even when I was asking her to work ninety days in a row. Literally. Her passion and commitment helped infuse this book with integrity.

I've known I wanted to write this book for a decade. My dear friend and colleague, Kirsten Collins, and I were at a spiritual retreat four years ago and I was seconds away from giving up for good. I was living in terror and victimhood—*Why can other people write and I can't? Maybe I just shouldn't try*. Kirsten bravely called me out, "If anyone has something to say, Molly, it's you: *What's going on?*" Good question. What *was* stopping me? And with that call to action I painstakingly went to work. Peeling off layers of fear and shame, I worked my tail off to get myself into emotional and spiritual shape to write this book with the truth and dignity that it deserved. Thank you, Kir, for believing in me in the best ways possible and for being the best hanai around.

I am a therapist who had to learn how to be an author. Big thanks to Linda Sivertsen and Will Lippincott, who taught me these ropes really quickly, and to Lisa Kaufmann, who met me where they left off and helped transform my vision into a fabulous proposal. Thank you to my "auntie" Lane Harkins, who was down for a read-through, an edit, or a teary call at the drop of a hat; to Laurel Mercer and Britta Barlogie, who excitingly and lovingly supported, brainstormed, and drafted with me until we were blue in the face. Thank you to those who graciously beta tested this book with speed, love, and fierce commitment to the cause: Erinn S, Ali L, Gail F, Robin G, Abby L, Gina P, Ben G, Karyn G, Ethan K, Michele L, and Michele S. Also, thank you to Google Docs, Google Scholar, and thesaurus.com—an author's real BFFs.

This book would never have come to fruition without Beacon Program, my clinic in Manhattan, and, as my mother would say, her first grandchild. It's where I was able to fine-tune all of my sometimes-wacky ideas, and where all of the concepts for this book were birthed. Beacon and I have been blessed with angels. People who walk in right when I need them and help me to take Beacon and our devoted mission and vision to the next level: Dan Shapiro, who constantly adds wisdom, guidance and grounding to my life in ways big and small; Strauss Zelnick, who helped me pick up the pieces when I was about to throw in the towel; Wendy Harris, my devoted supervisor and friend; Matt Arizin, who walked into Beacon one day when I had no one and stayed until I felt better; Elizabeth Fagan, Beacon's godmother; Andre Ivanoff, whom I'm blessed to have as a mentor; Scott Cannold, who provided me with a crash course in business; Scott Levy, who helped me make a business plan on five pieces of paper; and Rob Jackson and Pam Gold.

A huge debt of gratitude for Amorette Rojas, my longtime assistant, office manager, and "Molly whisperer," for her infinite love and dedication to me and Beacon, and to my incredible team, whom I cherish more than they can ever know: Kirsten Collins, Britta Barlogie, Laurel Mercer, Alex Wilt, and Teresa Vella. Thank you to Kate Metzler, Zulma Rodriguez, Gabrielle Breslow, Jaime Oliver, and Rachel Potter.

Most especially, thank you to the brave and courageous clients we get to treat, who allow us into their hearts and souls; to you I am forever indebted.

Thank you to my mentors, teachers, and colleagues through the years who have molded me into who I am today—some I know, some I don't, and all I love: Marsha Linehan, Ryan Craig, Diane Mickley, Caroline Myss, Tara Brach, Brené Brown, Andre Ivanoff, Marty Lerner, Wendy Harris, Charlie Swenson, Alan Fruzzetti, Alec Miller, Jill Rathus, Adam Carmel, Robert Lustig, Ashley Gearhardt, Nicole Avena, Joan Ilfland, Susan Pierce-Thompson, Dan Kirschenbaum, Brad Reedy, Tony Sparber, Elizabeth Gilbert, Glennon Doyle, Michael O'Brien, Evan Rofheart, Katherine Hamer, Rob Wergin, and Maritza Molina.

Thank you to my incredible spiritual community. You quite literally loved me until I could learn to love myself and helped me to develop the most important relationship in my life—one with a Higher Power. You are the most amazing humans I have ever met. You have taught me what connection, altruism, and communion is all about. Thank you to all of my fellows at 7:30 City Group, 4:45 Hope, 4:30 West Side, and the 79th Street Workshop. Thank you to my trusted guides: Kathleen McFeeters, Yara S, Rosemary Duffy, Kevin Talty, Shoshana Ostberg, Martha, Francesca M-A, Alan Schein, and Kathy Ashworth.

I have a depth in my friendships that has led me to coin the term "FRamily"— friends who are family. To my TRIBE who have lovingly welcomed my late-night-early-morning-hysterical-crying-I-really-just-can't calls, texts, dinner dates, stoop talks, and the like, and who are never *ever* surprised when all of these amazing things happen. To Erin Sitaris, my spiritual sister for preaching the truth and walking the path with me; to Alison Leipzig for taking my food, honoring my feelings, and sharing her creativity; and to the rest of my TRIBE. You incredible people have given the truest of definition to the term *Power Circle*: Dria DeBotton, Kirsten Collins, Stephanie Rudnick, Kristen Johnson, Elizabeth Fagan, Michelle Garside, Stephanie Tade, Britta Barlogie, Anne Wright, Heather Lasnier, Erin Jacques, Stefanie Eris, Jennifer Tannenbaum, Kimberly Moore, Samantha Smith, Jackie Schmidt, Adam Lelonek, Brad Lamm, Scott Levy, and Josh Wolfe.

I'm beyond grateful to my best friend and female soul mate, Michele Stocknoff, who can see the pinnacle far before my eye can even focus. She's fearlessly and generously showed me love and support through *literal* thick and thin—guiding me, believing in me, and reminding me that I'm never alone— with an easy *We got this, Moo!* I also have the deepest appreciation for Lauren Taylor Wolfe, my true ride-or-die sister who has always been able to see my best—especially when I can't. She has been an undying source of encouragement, love and comfort, has taught me what loyalty truly means . . . and how to dance at the late age of eighteen.

And thank you to my beloved godchildren: Ashton, Arianna, Carson, Quinn, and Bodhi, who have taught me a whole new definition of love.

Thank you to my family: my mom, Robin, who has always loved and sacrificed for me in ways big and small. I love you more than I can ever explain in words. Thank you to my stepfather, Alan, who has been the most relentless, mushiest cheerleader around; to my father, Jeff, whose legacy I am grateful to have connected to, and in the process, helped heal; my brothers and sister-in-law: Kevin, Mikey, and Rachel, who are always there making me laugh harder than anyone I know; Jennifer Corwin, a steadfast part of my foundation—my best friend since I was five, which makes her my family. The biggest thank-you to my cousins: Adam Carmel, Katie Azavedo, and Leigh-Ann Gluck, who have truly taught me what it means to have a family connection and who are also three of my very best friends.

And I know I've thanked you, my reader, about a zillion times. But just one more—thank you for picking up this book and considering my words and this solution. Please know that I am rooting for your success with the deepest of love and appreciation in my heart, always.

Notes

Chapter 3: The Truth About Your Sweetest Love

page 34   **trouble sleeping:** St-Onge, Marie-Pierre, Amy Roberts, Ari Shechter, and Arindam Roy Choudhury. "Fiber and saturated fat are associated with sleep arousals and slow wave sleep." *Journal of Clinical Sleep Medicine* 12, no. 1 (2016): 19–24.

page 34   **heart disease:** Yang, Quanhe, Zefeng Zhang, Edward W. Gregg, W. Dana Flanders, Robert Merritt, and Frank B. Hu. "Added sugar intake and cardiovascular diseases mortality among US adults." *JAMA Internal Medicine* 174, no. 4 (2014): 516–24.

page 34   **increased cholesterol:** Kelley, Glen L., Geoffrey Allan, and Salman Azhar. "High dietary fructose induces a hepatic stress response resulting in cholesterol and lipid dysregulation." *Endocrinology* 145, no. 2 (2004): 548–55.

page 34   **nonalcoholic fatty liver:** Clark, Jeanne M. "The epidemiology of nonalcoholic fatty liver disease in adults." *Journal of Clinical Gastroenterology* 40, suppl. 1 (2006): S5–10.

page 34   **leptin resistance:** Spreadbury, Ian. "Comparison with ancestral diets suggests dense acellular carbohydrates promote an inflammatory microbiota, and may be the primary dietary cause of leptin resistance and obesity." *Diabetes, Metabolic Syndrome and Obesity: Targets and Therapy* 5 (2012): 175–89.

page 34   **Sugar increases the risk of developing certain cancers:** Galeone, Carlotta, Claudio Pelucchi, and Carlo La Vecchia. "Added sugar, glycemic index and load in colon cancer risk." *Current Opinion in Clinical Nutrition & Metabolic Care* 15, no. 4 (2012): 368–73.

      Hodge, Allison M., Julie K. Bassett, Roger L. Milne, Dallas R. English, and Graham G. Giles. "Consumption of sugar-sweetened and artificially sweetened soft drinks and risk of obesity-related cancers." *Public Health Nutrition* 21, no. 9 (2018): 1618–26.

page 34 **glucose intolerance and diabetes:** Stanhope, Kimber L. "Sugar consumption, metabolic disease and obesity: The state of the controversy." *Critical Reviews in Clinical Laboratory Sciences* 53, no. 1 (2016): 52–67.

page 34 **when we ingest Sugar:** Lyssiotis, Costas A. and Lewis C. Cantley. "Metabolic syndrome: F stands for fructose and fat." *Nature* 502, no. 7470 (2013): 181.

page 36 **the obesity rate has quadrupled:** Johnson, Richard J., Mark S. Segal, Yuri Sautin, Takahiko Nakagawa, Daniel I. Feig, Duk-Hee Kang, Michael S. Gersch, Steven Benner, and Laura G. Sánchez-Lozada. "Potential role of sugar (fructose) in the epidemic of hypertension, obesity and the metabolic syndrome, diabetes, kidney disease, and cardiovascular disease." *American Journal of Clinical Nutrition* 86, no. 4 (2007): 899–906.

page 37 **greater desire and craving:** Greer, Stephanie M., Andrea N. Goldstein, and Matthew P. Walker. "The impact of sleep deprivation on food desire in the human brain." *Nature Communications* 4 (2013): 2259.

page 37 **more pleasurable:** St-Onge, M. P., S. Wolfe, M. Sy, A. Shechter, and J. Hirsch. "Sleep restriction increases the neuronal response to unhealthy food in normal-weight individuals." *International Journal of Obesity* 38, no. 3 (2014): 411–6.

page 37 **stressed we eat more:** Newman, Emily, Daryl B. O'Connor, and Mark Conner. "Daily hassles and eating behaviour: The role of cortisol reactivity status." *Psychoneuroendocrinology* 32, no. 2 (2007): 125–32.

page 37 **inevitably gain weight:** Torres, Susan J., and Caryl A. Nowson. "Relationship between stress, eating behavior, and obesity." *Nutrition* 23, no. 11–12 (2007): 887–94.

page 37 **It's the high-Sugar foods:** Epel, Elissa, Rachel Lapidus, Bruce McEwen, and Kelly Brownell. "Stress may add bite to appetite in women: A laboratory study of stress-induced cortisol and eating behavior." *Psychoneuroendocrinology* 26, no. 1 (2001): 37–49.

page 37 **counteract our stress response and boost our mood:** Markus, Rob, Geert Panhuysen, Adriaan Tuiten, and Hans Koppeschaar. "Effects of food on cortisol and mood in vulnerable subjects under controllable and uncontrollable stress." *Physiology & Behavior* 70, no. 3–4 (2000): 333–42.

page 38 **We use it constantly throughout the day:** Baumeister, Roy F., and John Tierney. *Willpower: Rediscovering the greatest human strength.* New York: Penguin, 2012.

page 38 **Tolerance . . . continued use despite negative consequences:** American Psychiatric Association. *Diagnostic and statistical manual of mental disorders (DSM-5).* Washington, DC: American Psychiatric Publishing, 2013.

page 39 **Responded to excessive Sugar intake with . . . withdrawal:** Colantuoni, Carlo, Pedro Rada, Joseph McCarthy, Caroline Patten, Nicole M. Avena, Andrew Chadeayne, and Bartley G. Hoebel. "Evidence that intermittent, excessive sugar intake causes endogenous opioid dependence." *Obesity Research* 10, no. 6 (2002): 478–88.

page 39 **nicotine withdrawal:** Wideman, C. H., G. R. Nadzam, and H. M. Murphy. "Implications of an animal model of sugar addiction, withdrawal and relapse for human health." *Nutritional Neuroscience* 8, no. 5–6 (2005): 269–76.

page 39 **less likely to swim or climb out, and more likely to passively float:** Avena, Nicole M., Pedro Rada, and Bartley G. Hoebel. "Evidence for sugar addiction: Behavioral and neurochemical effects of intermittent, excessive sugar intake." *Neuroscience & Biobehavioral Reviews* 32, no. 1 (2008): 20–39.

page 40 **start *storing* fat:** Kersten, Sander. "Mechanisms of nutritional and hormonal regulation of lipogenesis." *EMBO Reports* 2, no. 4 (2001): 282–6.

page 41 **breaks down the cell structure of the grain:** Venn, B. J., and J. I. Mann. "Cereal grains, legumes and diabetes." *European Journal of Clinical Nutrition* 58, no. 11 (2004): 1443–61.

page 41 **GI of about 68:** Foster-Powell, Kaye, Susanna H. A. Holt, and Janette C. Brand-Miller. "International table of glycemic index and glycemic load values: 2002." *American Journal of Clinical Nutrition* 76, no. 1 (2002): 5–56.

page 41 **more likely to report addictive eating:** Schulte, Erica M., Nicole M. Avena, and Ashley N. Gearhardt. "Which foods may be addictive? The roles of processing, fat content, and glycemic load." *PloS One* 10, no. 2 (2015): e0117959.

page 41 **increase reported hunger while stimulating brain regions:** Lennerz, Belinda S., David C. Alsop, Laura M. Holsen, Emily Stern, Rafael Rojas, Cara B. Ebbeling, Jill M. Goldstein, and David S. Ludwig. "Effects of dietary glycemic index on brain regions related to reward and craving in men." *American Journal of Clinical Nutrition* 98, no. 3 (2013): 641–7.

page 41 **white bread (GI 70) and baguettes (GI 95):** Foster-Powell, Holt, and Brand-Miller. "International table of glycemic index."

page 41 **strips away many of the essential nutrients and minerals:** Pedersen, Birthe, and B. O. Eggum. "The influence of milling on the nutritive value of flour from cereal grains. 2. Wheat." *Plant Foods for Human Nutrition* 33, no. 1 (1983): 51–61.

page 41   **removes the bran and germ:** Dewettinck, Koen, Filip Van Bockstaele, Bianka Kühne, Davy Van de Walle, T. M. Courtens, and Xavier Gellynck. "Nutritional value of bread: Influence of processing, food interaction and consumer perception." *Journal of Cereal Science* 48, no. 2 (2008): 243–57.

page 41   **wheat flour had only 30 percent of the minerals:** Pedersen, Birthe, and Eggum. "The influence of milling on the nutritive value of flour from cereal grains. 2. Wheat."

page 41   **digested far more quickly:** Venn and Mann. "Cereal grains, legumes and diabetes."

page 41   **rise in insulin levels:** Heaton, Kenneth W., S. N. Marcus, P. M. Emmett, and C. H. Bolton. "Particle size of wheat, maize, and oat test meals: Effects on plasma glucose and insulin responses and on the rate of starch digestion in vitro." *American Journal of Clinical Nutrition* 47, no. 4 (1988): 675–82.

page 41   **decrease in your ability to feel full when you're eating fiber:** Isaksson, Hanna, Birgitta Sundberg, Per Åman, Helena Fredriksson, and Johan Olsson. "Whole grain rye porridge breakfast improves satiety compared to refined wheat bread breakfast." *Food & Nutrition Research* 52 (2008).

page 43   **reward, and impulse-control systems:** Weinstein, Aviv, and Michel Lejoyeux. "New developments on the neurobiological and pharma co-genetic mechanisms underlying internet and videogame addiction." *American Journal on Addictions* 24, no. 2 (2015): 117–25.

     Potenza, Marc N. "Should addictive disorders include non-substance-related conditions?" *Addiction* 101, suppl. 1 (2006): 142–51.

page 43   **in the same way as substance addictions:** Han, Doug Hyun, Yang Soo Kim, Yong Sik Lee, Kyung Joon Min, and Perry F. Renshaw. "Changes in cue-induced, prefrontal cortex activity with video-game play." *Cyberpsychology, Behavior and Social Networking* 13, no. 6 (2010): 655–61.

page 44   **These same genes are found:** Smith, Dana G., and Trevor W. Robbins. "The neurobiological underpinnings of obesity and binge eating: A rationale for adopting the food addiction model." *Biological Psychiatry* 73, no. 9 (2013): 804–10.

page 44   **difficulty regulating your emotions:** Ducci, Francesca, and David Goldman. "Genetic approaches to addiction: Genes and alcohol." *Addiction* 103, no. 9 (2008): 1414–28.

page 44   **more impulsive:** Verdejo-García, Antonio, Andrew J. Lawrence, and
Luke Clark. "Impulsivity as a vulnerability marker for substance-use
disorders: Review of findings from high-risk research, problem
gamblers and genetic association studies." *Neuroscience &
Biobehavioral Reviews* 32, no. 4 (2008): 777–810.

      Bowirrat, Abdalla, and Marlene Oscar-Berman. "Relationship
between dopaminergic neurotransmission, alcoholism, and Reward
Deficiency syndrome." *American Journal of Medical Genetics Part B:
Neuropsychiatric Genetics* 132B, no. 1 (2005): 29–37.

page 44   **those with post-traumatic stress disorder (PTSD) rated higher:**
Mason, Susan M., Alan J. Flint, Andrea L. Roberts, Jessica Agnew-
Blais, Karestan C. Koenen, and Janet W. Rich-Edwards.
"Posttraumatic stress disorder symptoms and food addiction in
women by timing and type of trauma exposure." *JAMA Psychiatry*
71, no. 11 (2014): 1271–8.

page 44   **linked to food addiction, binge eating, and other dysfunctional:**
Imperatori, Claudio, Marco Innamorati, Dorian A. Lamis, Benedetto
Farina, Maurizio Pompili, Anna Contardi, and Mariantonietta
Fabbricatore. "Childhood trauma in obese and overweight women
with food addiction and clinical-level of binge eating." *Child Abuse &
Neglect* 58 (2016): 180–90.

Chapter 4: Defining Your Relationship

page 50   **The Yale Food Addiction Scale (YFAS):** Schulte, Erica M., and Ashley
N. Gearhardt. "Development of the modified Yale Food Addiction
Scale version 2.0." *European Eating Disorders Review* 25, no. 4
(2017): 302–8.

page 58   **greater chance of shortening the episode and preventing relapse:** US
Department of Health and Human Services. *Facing addiction in
America: The Surgeon General's report on alcohol, drugs, and
health.* Washington, DC: US Department of Health and Human
Services, 2016, 6.

Chapter 5: Don't Believe Everything You Think

page 69   **quicker to *act* your way into better habits:** Breuning, Loretta
Graziano. *Habits of a happy brain: Retrain your brain to boost your
serotonin, dopamine, oxytocin, & endorphin levels.* New York:
Simon & Schuster, 2015.

page 69   ***actions,* not thoughts, is responsible for forming new neural pathways
in our brain:** Ibid.

page 69   **those neural pathways . . . are what control and strengthen new
behaviors:** Everitt, Barry J., and Trevor W. Robbins. "Neural systems

of reinforcement for drug addiction: From actions to habits to compulsion." *Nature Neuroscience* 8, no. 11 (2005): 1481–9.

Chapter 6: Your 66-Day Vows

page 79   **six hundred times sweeter:** Center for Food Safety and Applied Nutrition. "Food additives & ingredients—additional information about high-intensity sweeteners permitted for use in food in the United States." US Food and Drug Administration, February 8, 2018. https://www.fda.gov/food/ingredientspackaginglabeling/food additivesingredients/ucm397725.htm.

page 79   **thirty times sweeter:** Goyal, S. K., Samsher, and R. K. Goyal. "Stevia (Stevia rebaudiana) a bio-sweetener: A review." *International Journal of Food Sciences and Nutrition* 61, no. 1 (2010): 1–10.

page 79   **three hundred times sweeter:** "Import Alert 45-06." US Food and Drug Administration, September 18, 2008. https://www.accessdata .fda.gov/cms_ia/importalert_119.html.

page 79   **artificial sweetener raises body mass index:** Stellman, Steven D., and Lawrence Garfinkel. "Artificial sweetener use and one-year weight change among women." *Preventive Medicine* 15, no. 2 (1986): 195–202.

　　　Blum, Janet Whatley, Dennis J. Jacobsen, and Joseph E. Donnelly. "Beverage consumption patterns in elementary school aged children across a two-year period." *Journal of the American College of Nutrition* 24, no. 2 (2005): 93–8.

page 80   **with a 47 percent increase in BMI:** Fowler, Sharon P., Ken Williams, Roy G. Resendez, Kelly J. Hunt, Helen P. Hazuda, and Michael P. Stern. "Fueling the obesity epidemic? Artificially sweetened beverage use and long-term weight gain." *Obesity* 16, no. 8 (2008): 1894–900.

page 80   **rats who were given artificial sweetener ate and weighed more:** Swithers, Susan E., and Terry L. Davidson. "A role for sweet taste: Calorie predictive relations in energy regulation by rats." *Behavioral Neuroscience* 122, no. 1 (2008): 161–73.

page 80   **artificial sweeteners enhance appetite and hunger:** Yang, Qing. "Gain weight by 'going diet?' Artificial sweeteners and the neurobiology of sugar cravings: Neuroscience 2010." *Yale Journal of Biology and Medicine* 83, no. 2 (2010): 101–8.

page 80   **Artificial sweetener affects your glycemic and insulin responses:** Pepino, M. Yanina, Courtney D. Tiemann, Bruce W. Patterson, Burton M. Wice, and Samuel Klein. "Sucralose affects glycemic and hormonal responses to an oral glucose load." *Diabetes Care* 36, no. 9 (2013): 2530–5.

page 80   **change gut bacteria, causing glucose intolerance:** Suez, Jotham, Tal Korem, David Zeevi, Gili Zilberman-Schapira, Christoph A. Thaiss,

Ori Maza, David Israeli et al. "Artificial sweeteners induce glucose intolerance by altering the gut microbiota." *Nature* 514, no. 7521 (2014): 181–6.

page 81   **students who chewed their lunch for longer had less snacking:** Higgs, Suzanne, and Alison Jones. "Prolonged chewing at lunch decreases later snack intake." *Appetite* 62 (2013): 91–5.

page 81   **chewing more can reduce food intake:** Smit, Hendrik Jan, E. Katherine Kemsley, Henri S. Tapp, and C. Jeya Henry. "Does prolonged chewing reduce food intake? Fletcherism revisited." *Appetite* 57, no. 1 (2011): 295–8.

Li, Jie, Na Zhang, Lizhen Hu, Ze Li, Rui Li, Cong Li, and Shuran Wang. "Improvement in chewing activity reduces energy intake in one meal and modulates plasma gut hormone concentrations in obese and lean young Chinese men." *American Journal of Clinical Nutrition* 94, no. 3 (2011): 709–16.

Andrade, Ana M., Geoffrey W. Greene, and Kathleen J. Melanson. "Eating slowly led to decreases in energy intake within meals in healthy women." *Journal of the American Dietetic Association* 108, no. 7 (2008): 1186–91.

page 81   **lower hunger, and increase fullness:** Cassady, Bridget A., James H. Hollis, Angie D. Fulford, Robert V. Considine, and Richard D. Mattes. "Mastication of almonds: Effects of lipid bioaccessibility, appetite, and hormone response." *American Journal of Clinical Nutrition* 89, no. 3 (2009): 794–800.

page 82   **drinking your Sugar makes you more prone to blood sugar crashes:** Haber, G. B., K. W. Heaton, D. Murphy, and L. F. Burroughs. "Depletion and disruption of dietary fibre. Effects on satiety, plasma-glucose, and serum-insulin." *Lancet* 310, no. 8040 (1977): 679–82.

page 84   **External cues like a TV:** Wansink, Brian, Collin R. Payne, and Pierre Chandon. "Internal and external cues of meal cessation: The French paradox redux?" *Obesity* 15, no. 12 (2007): 2920–4.

Shimizu, Mitsuru, and Brian Wansink. "Watching food-related television increases caloric intake in restrained eaters." *Appetite* 57, no. 3 (2011): 661–4.

page 85   **supersized containers, and large portion sizes:** Wansink, Brian, James E. Painter, and Jill North. "Bottomless bowls: Why visual cues of portion size may influence intake." *Obesity Research* 13, no. 1 (2005): 93–100.

page 85   **underestimate the number of food-related decisions we make:** Wansink, Brian, and Jeffery Sobal. "Mindless eating: The 200 daily food decisions we overlook." *Environment and Behavior* 39, no. 1 (2007): 106–23.

page 84　**The more distracted we are by them, the more mindlessly we eat:** Tal, Aner, Brian Wansink, and Scott Zuckerman. "Level of TV distraction influences amount eaten (626.20)." *FASEB Journal* 28, no. 1 supplement (2014).

page 86　**people who struggle with their weight snack frequently:** Kern, Lee S., Kelli E. Friedman, Simona K. Reichmann, Philip R. Costanzo, and Gerard J. Musante. "Changing eating behavior: A preliminary study to consider broader measures of weight control treatment success." *Eating Behaviors* 3, no. 2 (2002): 113–21.

page 86　**greater risk of weight gain:** van der Heijden, Amber Awa, Frank B. Hu, Eric B. Rimm, and Rob M. van Dam. "A prospective study of breakfast consumption and weight gain among U.S. men." *Obesity* 15, no. 10 (2007): 2463–9.

page 86　**type 2 diabetes:** Mekary, Rania A., Edward Giovannucci, Walter C. Willett, Rob M. van Dam, and Frank B. Hu. "Eating patterns and type 2 diabetes risk in men: Breakfast omission, eating frequency, and snacking." *American Journal of Clinical Nutrition* 95, no. 5 (2012): 1182–9.

page 86　**increased sensitivity to sweet taste:** Ninomiya, Yuzo, Noriatsu Shigemura, Keiko Yasumatsu, Rie Ohta, Kumiko Sugimoto, Kiyohito Nakashima, and Bernd Lindemann. "Leptin and sweet taste." *Vitamins and Hormones* 64 (2002): 221–48.

page 86　**waiting too long to eat . . . makes it more difficult to control your body weight:** Garaulet, Marta, Purificación Gómez-Abellán, Juan J. Alburquerque-Béjar, Yu-Chi Lee, Jose M. Ordovás, and Frank A. J. L. Scheer. "Timing of food intake predicts weight loss effectiveness." *International Journal of Obesity* 37, no. 4 (2013): 604–11.

　　Van Lippevelde, Wendy, Saskia J. Te Velde, Maïté Verloigne, Maartje M. Van Stralen, Ilse De Bourdeaudhuij, Yannis Manios, Elling Bere et al. "Associations between family-related factors, breakfast consumption and BMI among 10- to 12-year-old European children: The cross-sectional ENERGY-study." *PLoS One* 8, no. 11 (2013): e79550.

　　Timlin, Maureen T., Mark A. Pereira, Mary Story, and Dianne Neumark-Sztainer. "Breakfast eating and weight change in a 5-year prospective analysis of adolescents: Project EAT (Eating Among Teens)." *Pediatrics* 121, no. 3 (2008): e638–45.

　　Deshmukh-Taskar, P. R., T. A. Nicklas, C. E. O'Neil, D. R. Keast, J. D. Radcliffe, and S. Cho. "The relationship of breakfast skipping and type of breakfast consumption with nutrient intake and weight status in children and adolescents: The National Health and Nutrition

Examination Survey 1999–2006." *Journal of the American Dietetic Association* 110, no. 6 (2010): 869–78.

Szajewska, Hania, and Marek Ruszczynski. "Systematic review demonstrating that breakfast consumption influences body weight outcomes in children and adolescents in Europe." *Critical Reviews in Food Science and Nutrition* 50, no. 2 (2010): 113–9.

Berg, Christina, Georgios Lappas, Alicja Wolk, Elisabeth Strandhagen, Kjell Torén, Annika Rosengren, Dag Thelle, and Lauren Lissner. "Eating patterns and portion size associated with obesity in a Swedish population." *Appetite* 52, no. 1 (2009): 21–6.

Timlin, Pereira, Story et al. "Breakfast eating and weight change in a 5-year prospective analysis of adolescents."

page 86   **learn hunger with some consistent timing of meals:** Teff, Karen. "Learning hunger: conditioned anticipatory ghrelin responses in energy homeostasis." *Endocrinology* 147, no. 1 (2006): 20–22.

page 86   **With appropriate portions and consistent meals, you're less likely to overeat:** Brunstrom, Jeffrey M. "The control of meal size in human subjects: a role for expected satiety, expected satiation and premeal planning."*Proceedings of the Nutrition Society* 70, no. 2 (2011): 155–61.

page 87   **participants who set goals and planned:** Ziegelmann, Jochen P., and Sonia Lippke. "Planning and strategy use in health behavior change: A life span view." *International Journal of Behavioral Medicine* 14, no. 1 (2007): 30–9.

page 87   **Meal planning is associated with:** Ducrot, Pauline, Caroline Méjean, Vani Aroumougame, Gladys Ibanez, Benjamin Allès, Emmanuelle Kesse-Guyot, Serge Hercberg, and Sandrine Péneau. "Meal planning is associated with food variety, diet quality and body weight status in a large sample of French adults." *International Journal of Behavioral Nutrition and Physical Aactivity* 14, no. 1 (2017): 12.

page 88   **weighing regularly helps to release weight:** Linde, Jennifer A., Robert W. Jeffery, Simone A. French, Nicolaas P. Pronk, and Raymond G. Boyle. "Self-weighing in weight gain prevention and weight loss trials." *Annals of Behavioral Medicine* 30, no. 3 (2005): 210–6.

Butryn, Meghan L., Suzanne Phelan, James O. Hill, and Rena R. Wing. "Consistent self-monitoring of weight: A key component of successful weight loss maintenance." *Obesity* 15, no. 12 (2007): 3091–6.

Levitsky, D. A., J. Garay, M. Nausbaum, L. Neighbors, and D. M. Dellavalle. "Monitoring weight daily blocks the freshman weight gain: A model for combating the epidemic of obesity." *International Journal of Obesity* 30, no. 6 (2006): 1003–10.

page 88   **weighing too frequently is linked to unhealthy behaviors:** Neumark-Sztainer, Dianne, Patricia van den Berg, Peter J. Hannan, and Mary Story. "Self-weighing in adolescents: Helpful or harmful? Longitudinal associations with body weight changes and disordered eating." *Journal of Adolescent Health* 39, no. 6 (2006): 811–8.

page 88   **negative consequences on self-esteem, depression, and anxiety:** Ogden, Jane, and Catherine Whyman. "The effect of repeated weighing on psychological state." *European Eating Disorders Review* 5, no. 2 (1997): 121–30.

page 88   **spending too much time with the scale can have serious repercussions:** Klos, Lori A., Valerie E. Esser, and Molly M. Kessler. "To weigh or not to weigh: The relationship between self-weighing behavior and body image among adults." *Body Image* 9, no. 4 (2012): 551–4.

Chapter 7: Your Food Plan

page 97   **we've been led astray:** Malhotra, Aseem, Rita F. Redberg, and Pascal Meier. "Saturated fat does not clog the arteries: Coronary heart disease is a chronic inflammatory condition, the risk of which can be effectively reduced from healthy lifestyle interventions." *British Journal of Sports Medicine* 51, no. 15 (2017): 1111–2.

page 98   **fat actually sends the proper "stop" message:** Shapiro, Alexandra M., Nihal Tümer, Yongxin Gao, K. Y. Cheng, and Philip J. Scarpace. "Prevention and reversal of diet-induced leptin resistance with a sugar-free diet despite high fat content." *British Journal of Nutrition* 106, no. 3 (2011): 390–7.

page 98   **high fat *and* high Sugar:** Ibid.

page 98   **fat overconsumption to be linked to being overweight, even though Sugar:** Avena, Nicole M., Pedro Rada, and Bartley G. Hoebel. "Sugar and fat bingeing have notable differences in addictive-like behavior." *Journal of Nutrition* 139, no. 3 (2009): 623–8.

page 98   **makes an insulin-resistant person more prone to develop type 2 diabetes:** Brand-Miller, Janette C., Susanna H. A. Holt, Dorota B. Pawlak, and Joanna McMillan. "Glycemic index and obesity." *American Journal of Clinical Nutrition* 76, no. 1 (2002): 281S–5S.

page 105   **increase your appetite:** Page, Kathleen A., Owen Chan, Jagriti Arora, Renata Belfort-DeAguiar, James Dzuira, Brian Roehmholdt, Gary W. Cline et al. "Effects of fructose vs glucose on regional cerebral blood flow in brain regions involved with appetite and reward pathways." *JAMA* 309, no. 1 (2013): 63–70.

page 105   **cue your body to store weight:** Basciano, Heather, Lisa Federico, and Khosrow Adeli. "Fructose, insulin resistance, and metabolic dyslipidemia." *Nutrition & Metabolism* 2, no. 1 (2005): 5.

page 105 **increase feelings of fullness:** Paddon-Jones, Douglas, Eric Westman, Richard D. Mattes, Robert R. Wolfe, Arne Astrup, and Margriet Westerterp-Plantenga. "Protein, weight management, and satiety." *American Journal of Clinical Nutrition* 87, no. 5 (2008): 1558S–61S.

page 105 **promote weight loss:** Buchholz, Andrea C., and Dale A. Schoeller. "Is a calorie a calorie?" *American Journal of Clinical Nutrition* 79, no. 5 (2004): 899S–906S.

page 105 **eating fewer calories is a must in the weight-release game:** Westerterp, Klaas R. "Physical activity, food intake, and body weight regulation: Insights from doubly labeled water studies." *Nutrition Reviews* 68, no. 3 (2010): 148–54.

Chapter 8: Real Talk

page 118 **when we eat the foods we crave less frequently:** Myers, Candice A., Corby K. Martin, and John W. Apolzan. "Food cravings and body weight: a conditioning response." *Current Opinion in Endocrinology, Diabetes and Obesity* 25, no. 5 (2018): 298–302.

page 119 **meditation:** Tang, Yi-Yuan, Rongxiang Tang, and Michael I. Posner. "Mindfulness meditation improves emotion regulation and reduces drug abuse." *Drug and Alcohol Dependence* 163, suppl. 1 (2016): S13–8.

page 119 **strategies to decrease the duration and intensity of uncomfortable feelings:** Verduyn, Philippe, and Saskia Lavrijsen. "Which emotions last longest and why: The role of event importance and rumination." *Motivation and Emotion* 39, no. 1 (2015): 119–27.

page 119 **distracting:** Silvia, Paul J., and Jack W. Brehm. "Exploring alternative deterrents to emotional intensity: Anticipated happiness, distraction, and sadness." *Cognition and Emotion* 15, no. 5 (2001): 575–92.

page 122 **decrease their suicide attempts by 70 percent:** McCauley, Elizabeth, Michele S. Berk, Joan R. Asarnow, Molly Adrian, Judith Cohen, Kathyrn Korslund, Claudia Avina et al. "Efficacy of dialectical behavior therapy for adolescents at high risk for suicide: A randomized clinical trial." *JAMA Psychiatry* 75, no. 8 (2018): 777–85.

page 122 **whole host of other incredible outcomes:** Koons, Cedar R., Clive J. Robins, J. Lindsey Tweed, Thomas R. Lynch, Alicia M. Gonzalez, Jennifer Q. Morse, G. Kay Bishop, Marian I. Butterfield, and Lori A. Bastian. "Efficacy of dialectical behavior therapy in women veterans with borderline personality disorder." *Behavior Therapy* 32, no. 2 (2001): 371–90.

page 122 **for both addiction:** Dimeff, Linda A., and Marsha M. Linehan. "Dialectical behavior therapy for substance abusers." *Addiction Science & Clinical Practice* 4, no. 2 (2008): 39–47.

page 122 **eating disorders:** Telch, Christy F., W. Stewart Agras, and Marsha M. Linehan. "Dialectical behavior therapy for binge eating disorder." *Journal of Consulting and Clinical Psychology* 69, no. 6 (2001): 1061–5.

page 122 **this quote:** Linehan, Marsha. *DBT skills training manual*, 2nd ed. New York: Guilford Publications, 2014.

page 123 **helps you to tolerate the moment without making it worse:** Ibid.

Chapter 9: Filling That Gaping Hole

page 133 **better performance and success:** Omar-Fauzee, Mohd Sofian, Wan Rezawana Binti Wan Daud, Rahim Abdullah, and Salleh Abd Rashid. "The effectiveness of imagery and coping strategies in sport performance." *European Journal of Social Sciences* 9, no. 1 (2009): 97–108.

Omar Sadeghi, Hassan, Mohd Sofian Omar-Fauzee, Marjohan Jamalis, Rozita Ab-Latif, and Majid Chahrdah Cheric. "The mental skills training of university soccer players." *International Education Studies* 3, no. 2 (2010): 81–90.

page 135 **your breath and heart rate slow:** Linehan. *DBT skills training manual.*

page 136 **rats chose heroin over water far less frequently than those in isolation:** Hari, Johann. "Everything you think you know about addiction is wrong [TED Talk]." Bruno Giussani (Director). New York: TED (2015).

page 136 **defines connection as:** Brown, Brené. *The gifts of imperfection: Let go of who you think you're supposed to be and embrace who you are.* Center City, MN: Hazelden, 2010.

page 138 **higher satisfaction with life . . . stronger relationships:** Emmons, Richard A., and Michael E. McCullough. "Counting blessings versus burdens: Experimental studies of gratitude and subjective well-being." *Journal of Personality and Social Psychology* 84, no. 2 (2003): 377–89.

McCullough, Michael E., Robert A. Emmons, and Jo-Ann Tsang. "The grateful disposition: A conceptual and empirical topography." *Journal of Personality and Social Psychology* 82, no. 1 (2002): 112–27.

page 138 **able to cope with stressful life events . . . stronger relationships:** Emmons, Robert A., and Robin Stern. "Gratitude as a psychotherapeutic intervention." *Journal of Clinical Psychology* 69, no. 8 (2013): 846–55.

Emmons, Robert A., and Charles M. Shelton. "Gratitude and the science of positive psychology." In *Oxford handbook of positive psychology*, 2nd ed., edited by C. R. Snyder and S. J. Lopez, 459–71. New York: Oxford University Press, 2002.

page 138 **improving sleep and lessening your physical ailments:** Emmons and McCullough. "Counting blessings versus burdens."

page 138 **prayer . . . helps you experience more gratitude:** Lambert, Nathaniel M., Frank D. Fincham, Scott R. Braithwaite, Steven M. Graham, and Steven R. H. Beach. "Can prayer increase gratitude?" *Psychology of Religion and Spirituality* 1, no. 3 (2009): 139–49.

page 138 **meditation . . . helps you experience more gratitude:** Shapiro, Shauna L., Gary E. R. Schwartz, and Craig Santerre. "Meditation and positive psychology." In Snyder and Lopez, *Oxford handbook of positive psychology*, 632–45.

page 138 **prayer has been shown to decrease anxiety and depression:** Boelens, Peter A., Roy R. Reeves, William H. Replogle, and Harold G. Koenig. "A randomized trial of the effect of prayer on depression and anxiety." *International Journal of Psychiatry in Medicine* 39, no. 4 (2009): 377–92.

page 138 **increase immune system functioning:** Çoruh, Başak, Hana Ayele, Meredith Pugh, and Thomas Mulligan. "Does religious activity improve health outcomes? A critical review of the recent literature." *Explore: The Journal of Science and Healing* 1, no. 3 (2005): 186–91.

page 138 **enhance your self-control:** Friese, Malte, and Michaela Wänke. "Personal prayer buffers self-control depletion." *Journal of Experimental Social Psychology* 51 (2014): 56–9.

page 139 **regulate behavior, reduce stress, and keep your emotions steady— improving overall emotional health:** Keng, Shian-Ling, Moria J. Smoski, and Clive J. Robins. "Effects of mindfulness on psychological health: A review of empirical studies." *Clinical Psychology Review* 31, no. 6 (2011): 1041–56.

page 139 **reduce stress:** MacLean, Christopher R. K., Kenneth G. Walton, Stig R. Wenneberg, Debra K. Levitsky, Joseph P. Mandarino, Rafiq Waziri, Stephen L. Hillis, and Robert H. Schneider. "Effects of the Transcendental Meditation program on adaptive mechanisms: Changes in hormone levels and responses to stress after 4 months of practice." *Psychoneuroendocrinology* 22, no. 4 (1997): 277–95.

page 139 **improves physical health, strengthens the immune system:** Davidson, Richard J., Jon Kabat-Zinn, Jessica Schumacher, Melissa Rosenkranz, Daniel Muller, Saki F. Santorelli, Ferris Urbanowski, Anne Harrington, Katherine Bonus, and John F. Sheridan. "Alterations in brain and immune function produced by mindfulness meditation." *Psychosomatic Medicine* 65, no. 4 (2003): 564–70.

Ngô, Thanh-Lan. "Review of the effects of mindfulness meditation on mental and physical health and its mechanisms of action." *Santé Mentale au Québec* 38, no. 2 (2013): 19–34.

Gard, Tim, Britta K. Hölzel, and Sara W. Lazar. "The potential effects of meditation on age-related cognitive decline: A systematic review." *Annals of the New York Academy of Sciences* 1307, no. 1 (2014): 89–103.

page 139 **aids sleep:** Winbush, Nicole Y., Cynthia R. Gross, and Mary Jo Kreitzer. "The effects of mindfulness-based stress reduction on sleep disturbance: A systematic review." *Explore: The Journal of Science and Healing* 3, no. 6 (2007): 585–91.

page 139 **mindfulness can . . . reduce cravings:** Tapper, Katy. "Mindfulness and craving: Effects and mechanisms." *Clinical Psychology Review* 59 (2018): 101–17.

page 140 **isn't any data that shows that increased exercise *alone* helps:** Paravidino, Vitor Barreto, Mauro Felippe Felix Mediano, Daniel J. Hoffman, and Rosely Sichieri. "Effect of exercise intensity on spontaneous physical activity energy expenditure in overweight boys: A crossover study." *PloS One* 11, no. 1 (2016): e0147141.

page 140 **increasing your appetite, how much you eat:** Church, Timothy S., Corby K. Martin, Angela M. Thompson, Conrad P. Earnest, Catherine R. Mikus, and Steven N. Blair. "Changes in weight, waist circumference and compensatory responses with different doses of exercise among sedentary, overweight postmenopausal women." *PloS One* 4, no. 2 (2009): e4515.

page 140 **decrease stress and depression:** Hassmén, Peter, Nathalie Koivula, and Antti Uutela. "Physical exercise and psychological well-being: A population study in Finland." *Preventive Medicine* 30, no. 1 (2000): 17–25.

page 140 **physical impacts:** Reiner, Miriam, Christina Niermann, Darko Jekauc, and Alexander Woll. "Long-term health benefits of physical activity—a systematic review of longitudinal studies." *BMC Public Health* 13, no. 1 (2013): 813.

page 140 **reduce stress, increase attention, and decrease emotional reactivity:** Ma, Xiao, Zi-Qi Yue, Zhu-Qing Gong, Hong Zhang, Nai-Yue Duan, Yu-Tong Shi, Gao-Xia Wei, and You-Fa Li. "The effect of diaphragmatic breathing on attention, negative affect and stress in healthy adults." *Frontiers in Psychology* 8 (2017): 874.

page 140 **improved organ functioning:** Ritz, Thomas, and Walton T. Roth. "Behavioral interventions in asthma. Breathing training." *Behavior Modification* 27, no. 5 (2003): 710–30.

page 140 **reduced hypertension:** Anderson, David E., Beverly A. Parsons, Jessica C. McNeely, and Edgar R. Miller. "Salt sensitivity of blood pressure is accompanied by slow respiratory rate: Results of a clinical feeding study." *Journal of the American Society of Hypertension* 1, no. 4 (2007): 256–63.

page 140 **decreased pain:** Mehling, Wolf E., Kathryn A. Hamel, Michael Acree, Nancy Byl, and Frederick M. Hecht. "Randomized, controlled trial of breath therapy for patients with chronic low-back pain." *Alternative Therapies in Health and Medicine* 11, no. 4 (2005): 44–52.

Zautra, Alex J., Robert Fasman, Mary C. Davis, and A. D. Craig "The effects of slow breathing on affective responses to pain stimuli: An experimental study." *Pain* 149, no. 1 (2010): 12–8.

page 141 **less dopamine is released when you're eating food *and* when you're:** Volkow, Nora D., George F. Koob, and A. Thomas McLellan. "Neurobiologic advances from the brain disease model of addiction." *New England Journal of Medicine* 374, no. 4 (2016): 363–71.

page 141 **reward system will recover:** Ibid.

page 141 **brain releases dopamine, serotonin, and endorphins:** Dfarhud, Dariush, Maryam Malmir, and Mohammad Khanahmadi. "Happiness & health: The biological factors—Systematic review article." *Iranian Journal of Public Health* 43, no. 11 (2014): 1468–77.

page 141 **enhance your feelings of pleasure and block feelings of stress:** Berk, Lee S., and Stanley A. Tan. "[beta]-Endorphin and HGH increase are associated with both the anticipation and experience of mirthful laughter." *FASEB Journal* 20, no. 4 (2006): A382.

Sprouse-Blum, Adam S., Greg Smith, Daniel Sugai, and F. Don Parsa. "Understanding endorphins and their importance in pain management." *Hawaii Medical Journal* 69, no. 3 (2010): 70–1.

page 141 **improve your mood and decrease your feelings of sadness and depression:** Sin, Nancy L., and Sonja Lyubomirsky. "Enhancing well-being and alleviating depressive symptoms with positive psychology interventions: A practice-friendly meta-analysis." *Journal of Clinical Psychology* 65, no. 5 (2009): 467–87.

page 141 **Cultivating your creativity is one of the most useful and effective ways:** Brown. *The gifts of imperfection.*

Chapter 11: Purgatory

page 156 **Grief is commonly defined as:** James, J., and R. Friedman. *The grief recovery handbook, 20th anniversary expanded edition.* New York: HarperCollins, 2009.

page 157 **model that identifies five stages of grief:** Kübler-Ross, Elisabeth. *On death and dying.* London, UK: Routledge, 1973.

page 157 **can be experienced in any order, without any sort of timeline:** Maciejewski, Paul K., Baohui Zhang, Susan D. Block, and Holly G.

Prigerson. "An empirical examination of the stage theory of grief." *JAMA* 297, no. 7 (2007): 716–23.

page 159 described as the *what-if* and *if-only* stage: Kübler-Ross, Elisabeth, and David Kessler. "The five stages of grief." In *On grief and grieving*, number ed., 7–30. City: Publisher, 2009.

page 161 characterizes acceptance as: Prigerson, Holly G., and Paul K. Maciejewski. "Grief and acceptance as opposite sides of the same coin: Setting a research agenda to study peaceful acceptance of loss." *British Journal of Psychiatry* 193, no. 6 (2008): 435–7.

page 161 effects hold true regardless of whether someone believed the rituals: Norton, Michael I., and Francesca Gino. "Rituals alleviate grieving for loved ones, lovers, and lotteries." *Journal of Experimental Psychology: General* 143, no. 1 (2014): 266–72.

page 161 *type* of ritual you choose is not important; the key is simply to do it: Ibid.

page 162 stopping results in withdrawal symptoms: Avena, Rada, and Hoebel. "Evidence for sugar addiction."

Colantuoni, Rada, McCarthy et al. "Evidence that intermittent, excessive sugar intake causes endogenous opioid dependence."

Schulte, Erica M., Julia K. Smeal, Jessi Lewis, and Ashley N. Gearhardt. "Development of the highly processed food withdrawal scale." *Appetite* 131 (2018): 148–54.

Chapter 12: Finding Love Again

page 169 effective in both addiction recovery *and* weight loss: Ruiz, Francisco J. "A review of acceptance and commitment therapy (ACT) empirical evidence: Correlational, experimental psychopathology, component and outcome studies." *International Journal of Psychology and Psychological Therapy* 10, no. 1 (2010): 125–62.

page 169 they are less impulsive, more able to tolerate pain, and experience less discomfort: Ibid.

page 171 "He who has a Why to live for can bear almost any How: Nietzsche, Friedrich. "Twilight of the Idols: 'Maxims and Arrows'" (1892).

Chapter 13: Getting to Gray

page 179 calls this concept *dialectical abstinence*: Dimeff and Linehan. "Dialectical behavior therapy for substance abusers."

page 180 go for the gold: Linehan, Marsha. *DBT Skills training manual*. New York: Guilford Publications, 2014.

Chapter 14: Divorcing Dieting

page 192 Abusive relationships function the very same way: Morgan, Hillary J., and Phillip R. Shaver. "Attachment processes and commitment to romantic relationships." In *Handbook of interpersonal commitment and relationship stability*, edited by Warren H. Jones, 109–24. Boston: Springer, 1999.

page 193 **FOMO was coined:** Kozodoy, Peter. "The inventor of FOMO is warning leaders about a new, more dangerous threat." *Inc.*, October 9, 2017. https://www.inc.com/peter-kozodoy/inventor-of-fomo-is -warning-leaders-about-a-new-more-dangerous-threat.html.

page 193 **describes it as:** Przybylski, Andrew K., Kou Murayama, Cody R. DeHaan, and Valerie Gladwell. "Motivational, emotional, and behavioral correlates of fear of missing out." *Computers in Human Behavior* 29, no. 4 (2013): 1841–8.

page 193 **diet industry earning sixty-six billion dollars a year:** "The U.S. weight loss & diet control market." Marketdata, May 2017. https:// www.marketresearch.com/Marketdata-Enterprises-Inc-v416/Weight -Loss-Diet-Control-10825677/.

Chapter 15: Finding Freedom in Humble Eating

page 200 **motivation needs to come from *within you*:** Ryan, Richard M., and Edward L. Deci. "Self-determination theory and the facilitation of intrinsic motivation, social development, and well-being." *American Psychologist* 55, no. 1 (2000): 68–78.

Deci, Edward L., and Richard M. Ryan. "The 'what' and 'why' of goal pursuits: Human needs and the self-determination of behavior." *Psychological Inquiry* 11, no. 4 (2000): 227–68.

page 200 **you're more likely to change:** Ryan, R. M., H. Patrick, E. L. Deci, and G. C. Williams. "Facilitating health behaviour change and its maintenance: Interventions based on self-determination theory." *European Health Psychologist* 10, no. 1 (2008): 2–5.

page 200 **successful eating regulation:** Mata, J., M. N. Silva, P. N. Vieira, E. V. Carraça, A. M. Andrade, S. R. Coutinho, L. B. Sardinha, and P. J. Teixeira. "Motivational 'spill-over' during weight control: Increased self-determination and exercise intrinsic motivation predict eating self-regulation." *Health Psychology*, 28, no. 6 (2009): 709–16.

page 200 **increased physical activity, greater weight loss:** Silva, M. N., P. N. Vieira, S. R. Coutinho, C. S. Minderico, M. G. Matos, L. B. Sardinha, and P. J. Teixeira. "Using self-determination theory to promote physical activity and weight control: A randomized controlled trial in women." *Journal of Behavioral Medicine* 33, no. 2 (2010): 110–22.

page 200 **greater weight loss:** Williams, G. C., V. M. Grow, Z. R. Freedman, R. M. Ryan, and E. L. Deci. "Motivational predictors of weight loss and weight-loss maintenance." *Journal of Personality and Social Psychology* 70, no. 1 (1996): 115–26.

Index